Pathophysiology
for Nurses
at a Glance

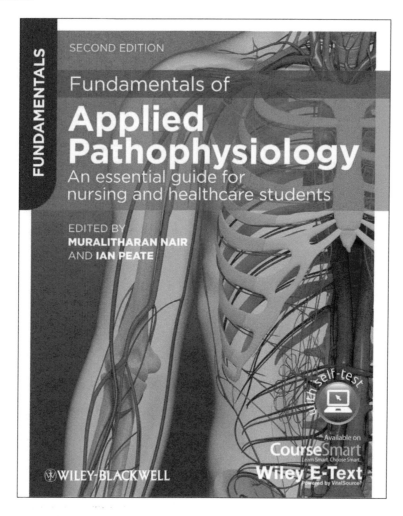

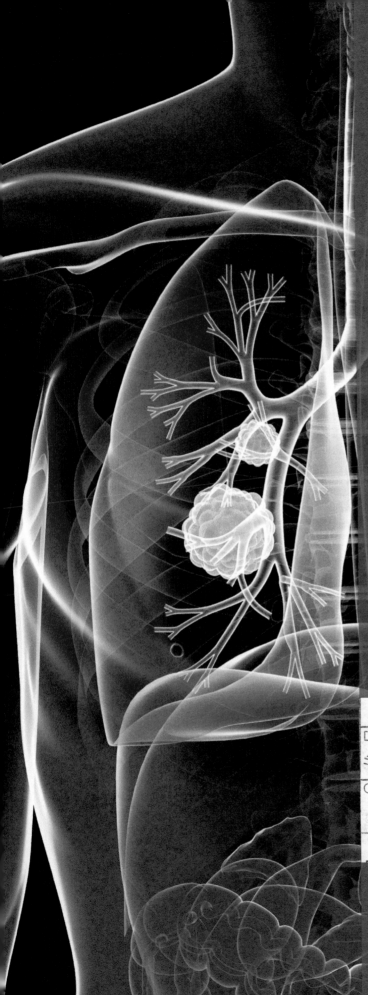

Pathophysiology for Nurses at a Glance

Muralitharan Nair
Independent Nursing Consultant
England

Ian Peate
Professor of Nursing
Head of School
School of Health Studies
Gibraltar

Series Editor: Ian Peate

WILEY Blackwell

Library of Congress Cataloging-in-Publication Data

Nair, Muralitharan, author.
Pathophysiology for nurses at a glance / Muralitharan Nair, Ian Peate.
    p. ; cm. – (At a glance series)
    Includes bibliographical references and index.
    ISBN 978-1-118-74606-6 (paper)
I. Peate, Ian, author.   II. Title.   III. Series: At a glance series (Oxford, England)
[DNLM: 1. Pathologic Processes–physiopathology–Nurses' Instruction.   2. Pathologic Processes–etiology–Nurses' Instruction.   QZ 140]
    RB127
    616′.047–dc23

                                        2014032709

A catalogue record for this book is available from the British Library.

Wiley also publishes its books in a variety of electronic formats. Some content that appears in print may not be available in electronic books.

Cover image: iStock / © Eraxion

Set in 9.5/11.5pt Minion by SPi Publisher Services, Pondicherry, India

Printed in the UK

Contents

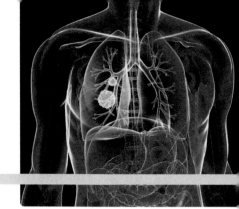

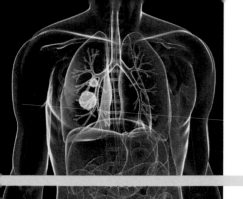

Preface

Pathophysiology for Nurses at a Glance provides you with a concise overview of a number health-related conditions. This text has been written with the intention of making the sometimes complex subject of pathophysiology understandable and stimulating. The human body has an astonishing capacity to respond to disease in a variety of physiological and psychological ways; it is able to compensate for the changes that occur caused by the disease process. This text considers those changes (the pathophysiological processes) and the effect they can have on a person.

Pathophysiology is concerned with the disturbance of normal mechanical, physical and biochemical functions. The word pathophysiology is a combined word from the Greek *pathos*, which means disease, and physiology is related to the numerous normal functions of the human body. Pathophysiology considers both the cellular and the organ changes that occur with disease, as well as the impact these changes have on body function. When something influences the normal physiological functioning of the body (such as disease), then this becomes a pathophysiological issue. It must be remembered, however, that normal health is not and cannot be exactly the same in any two people; as such, the term **normal** must be treated with caution.

To be able to care for people in a safe and effective manner, the nurse must have the knowledge and skills to meet needs inside and outside hospital and across health and social care, and meet the needs of an increasing older population and of those with long-term conditions.

This text is mainly intended for nursing students who will come into contact with those who may have a variety of physically related healthcare problems such as pneumonia, diabetes mellitus and many more diseases. The focus of the text is on the adult person.

It is the intention of this text to develop knowledge and skills both in theory and practice and to apply this knowledge with the intention of providing safe and effective high-quality care. The overriding aim is to relate normal body function to pathological changes that may lead to disease processes, preventing the individual from leading a 'normal' life.

Using the fundamental approach found in this will text will provide readers with an essential understanding of applied pathophysiology.

Muralitharan Nair
Ian Peate

Abbreviations

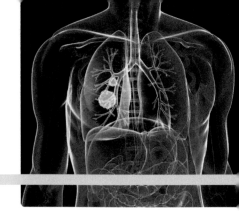

ABG	arterial blood gas	ESWL	extracorporeal shock wave lithotripsy
ACE	angiotensin-converting enzyme	FBC	full blood count
ADL	activities of daily living	Fe	iron
ALL	acute lymphoblastic leukaemia	FU	fluorouracil
AKI	acute kidney injury	GFR	glomerular filtration rate
AML	acute myeloid leukaemia	GH	growth hormone
AP resection	abdominoperineal resection	GI	gastrointestinal
ATN	acute tubular injury	GTN	glycerine trinitrate
ATRA	all trans retinoic acid	Hb	haemoglobin
AV	atrioventricular	HBV	hepatitis B virus
BBB	blood-brain barrier	HCC	hepatocellular cancer
BECA 2	BReast CAncer gene 2	HCL	hydrochloric acid
BMI	body mass index	HCO3	bicarbonate
BP	blood pressure	HCV	hepatitis C virus
BPH	benign prostatic hypertrophy	HIV	human immunodeficiency virus
BPM	beats per minute	*H Pylori*	*Helicobacter pylori*
BRCA 1	BReast CAncer gene 1	HUS	haemolytic-uremic syndrome
Ca	calcium	ICP	intracranial pressure
CB	chronic bronchitis	IDDM	insulin dependent diabetes mellitus
CBC	complete blood count	ITP	idiopathic thrombocytopenic purpura
CBF	cerebral blood flow	IV	intravenous
CCF	Congestive cardiac (heart) failure	IVC	inferior vena cava
CCU	cardiac care unit	K^+	potassium
CHD	coronary heart disease	LMWH	low molecular weight heparin
CKD	chronic kidney disease	mg	milligramme
Cl	chloride	MI	myocardial infarction
CLL	chronic lymphoblastic leukaemia	mL	millilitre
cm	centimetre	MS	multiple sclerosis
CML	chronic myeloid leukaemia	MSU	midstream specimen of urine
CO	cardiac output	MRI	magnetic resonance imaging
CO_2	carbon dioxide	Na	sodium
COPD	chronic obstructive pulmonary disease	NICE	National Institute for Health and Care Excellence
CSF	cerebrospinal fluid	NIDDM	non-insulin dependent diabetes mellitus
CTPA	computed tomography pulmonary angiogram	NIV	non-invasive ventilation
CVA	cerebrovascular accident	NSAID	non-steroidal anti-inflammatory drug
CVD	cardiovascular disease	O_2	oxygen
DNA	deoxyribonucleic acid	OA	osteoarthritis
DVT	deep vein thrombosis	PAD	peripheral arterial disease
ECG	elecrocardiograph	PEFR	peak expiratory flow rate
ECM	extracellular matrix	PE	pulmonary embolism
ED	erectile dysfunction	PD	Parkinson's disease
ER	endoplasmic reticulum	pH	measures of the acidity or alkalinity of a solution
ECSL	extracorporeal shockwave lithotripsy	PPI	proton pump inhibitors

PVD	peripheral vascular disease	TURBT	transurethral resection of bladder tumour
SA	sinoatrial	TURP	transurethral resection of the prostate
SOB	short of breath	UC	ulcerative colitis
SVC	superior vena cava	um	micrometre
TIA	transient ischaemic attack	UTI	urinary tract infection
TPN	total parenteral nutrition	VUR	vesicoureteral reflux
TTP	thrombotic thrombocytopenic purpura	WBC	white blood cells

Acknowledgements

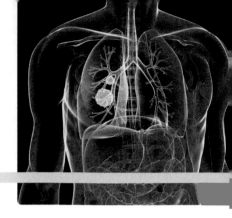

We acknowledge with thanks the use of material from other John Wiley & Sons publications:

Mehta, A. & Hoffbrand, V. (2014) *Haematology at a Glance*, 4e. John Wiley & Sons, Ltd, Oxford. Reproduced with permission of John Wiley & Sons, Ltd.

Peate, I. & Nair, M. (2011) *Fundamentals of Anatomy and Physiology for Student Nurses*. John Wiley & Sons, Ltd, Oxford. Reproduced with permission of John Wiley & Sons, Ltd.

Peate, I., Wild, K. & Nair, M. (eds) (2014) *Nursing Practice: Knowledge and Care*. John Wiley & Sons, Ltd, Oxford. Reproduced with permission of John Wiley & Sons, Ltd.

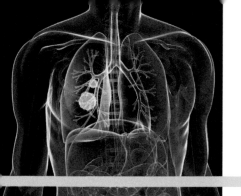

How to use your revision guide

Features contained within your revision guide

Each topic is presented in a double-page spread with clear, easy-to-follow diagrams supported by succinct explanatory text.

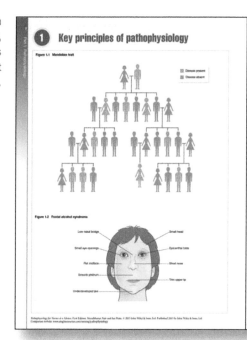

About the companion website

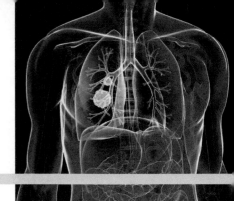

Don't forget to visit the companion website for this book:

**www.ataglanceseries.com/nursing/
pathophysiology**

There you will find valuable material designed to enhance
your learning, including:

- Interactive multiple-choice questions
- Case studies to test your knowledge

Scan this QR code to visit the companion website:

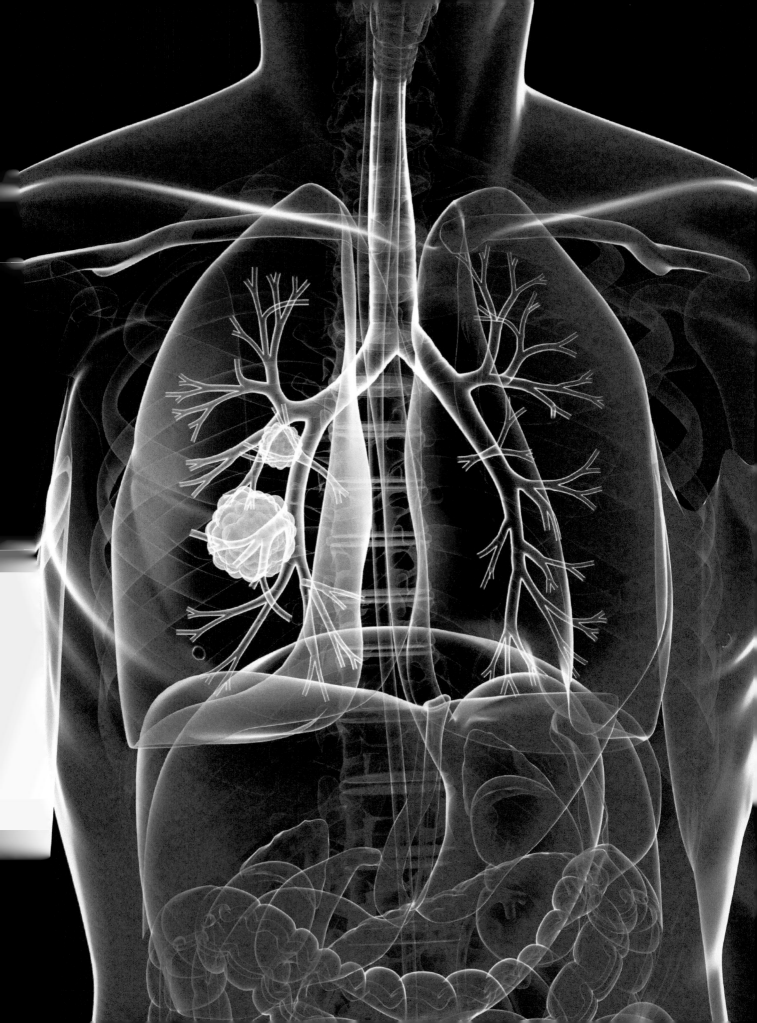

Pathophysiology

Part 1

Chapters

1 Key principles of pathophysiology

Figure 1.1 Mendelian trait

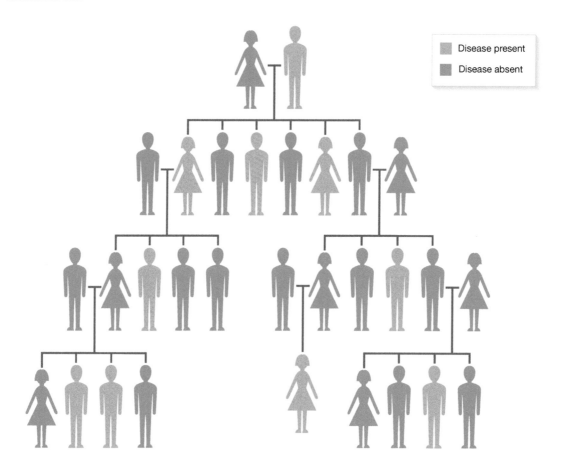

Disease present
Disease absent

Figure 1.2 Foetal alcohol syndrome

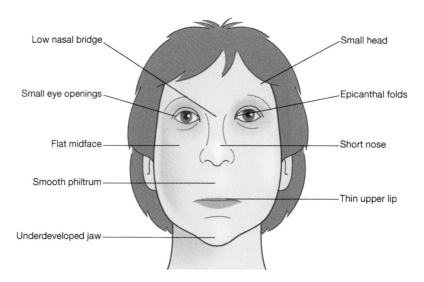

Low nasal bridge

Small eye openings

Flat midface

Smooth philtrum

Underdeveloped jaw

Small head

Epicanthal folds

Short nose

Thin upper lip

Pathophysiology for Nurses at a Glance, First Edition. Muralitharan Nair and Ian Peate. © 2015 John Wiley & Sons, Ltd. Published 2015 by John Wiley & Sons, Ltd.
Companion website: www.ataglanceseries.com/nursing/pathophysiology

Pathophysiology versus pathology

While both terms indicate the study of disease, the term pathology is a broader term dealing with all aspects of a disease. This study is valuable for a physician or a pathologist who is also interested in the macro and microscopic characteristics of tissues and organs. On the other hand, in pathophysiology the focus is on the abnormal function of diseased organs, with application to diagnostic procedures leading patient care. Healthcare professionals are more concerned with pathophysiology when dealing with patients.

Disease and aetiology

The study of the cause of disease is called aetiology. Aetiology is the preferred spelling in some countries, including the UK, whereas 'etiology' without an 'a' is used in the USA. The word 'aetiology' comes from the Greek *aitia*, cause + *logos*, discourse. Diseases are described as genetic, congenital or acquired.

Genetic

In a disease where the cause is genetic, the person may have a defective gene that causes the disease. These defective genes are often passed on to children by parents. These abnormalities can range from a small mutation in a single gene to the addition or subtraction of an entire chromosome or set of chromosomes.

Some genetic diseases are called Mendelian disorders (Figure 1.1); they are caused by mutations that occur in the DNA sequence of a single gene. These are usually rare diseases; some examples are Huntington's disease and cystic fibrosis. Many genetic diseases are multifactorial – they are caused by mutations in several genes, compounded by environmental factors. Some examples of these are heart disease, cancer and diabetes.

Congenital

In congenital disease, the genetic information is intact; however, problems with the intrauterine environment may result in congenital disorder. For example, cystic fibrosis is a genetic disorder, whereas foetal alcohol syndrome results from the mother's alcohol intake during pregnancy. This results in congenital abnormalities in a child who is genetically normal (Figure 1.2).

Acquired

In this type of disease, the person develops the disease after birth as a result of direct or indirect contact with another person or the environment. Examples include tuberculosis, emphysema, chicken pox or acquired heart diseases.

Signs and symptoms

A symptom is generally subjective, while a sign is objective. Any objective evidence of a disease, such as blood in the stool or a skin rash, is a sign – it can be recognized by the doctor, nurse, family members and the patient. However, stomachache, lower-back pain, fatigue, for example, can only be detected or sensed by the patient – others only know about it if the patient tells them. For example, pain can either be acute or chronic. An example of acute pain is abdominal pain, which is sudden and may last only a few hours or longer. Common chronic pain complaints include headache, low back pain, cancer pain, arthritis pain, neurogenic pain (pain resulting from damage to the peripheral nerves or to the central nervous system itself), psychogenic pain (pain not due to past disease or injury or any visible sign of damage inside or outside the nervous system).

Pathogenesis

In assessing a patient's signs and symptoms, conclusions can often be drawn about the pattern and development of a disease, in other words its pathogenesis. A typical pathogenesis involves kinds of tissue damage which produces certain effects. The progress of the disease can produce signs and symptoms throughout the course of the disease.

Another aspect of pathogenesis is the time over which the disease develops. Some may be acute, while others are chronic. Acute conditions have a rapid onset with short duration, while chronic conditions last for a longer period which could be from months to years.

Investigations and diagnosis

In order to make a diagnosis, it may be necessary to carry out some investigations to confirm the diagnosis. Some of the investigations may be invasive, while others are not invasive. These may include blood test, CT scans, chest X-rays, endoscopy and many more.

Diagnosis is identification of a condition, disease, disorder or problem by systematic analysis of the background or history, examination of the signs or symptoms, evaluation of the research or test results, and investigation of the assumed or probable causes. It is from the diagnosis that care or treatment is prescribed.

Treatment

Once a diagnosis is confirmed then the treatment can proceed. The treatment is either medical or nursing treatment. The aim of the treatment of a disease is to achieve a cure or minimize the patient's signs and symptoms to a degree where the patient can function near normality.

Prognosis

Prognosis is a prediction of the chance of recovery or survival from a disease. Most doctors give a prognosis based on statistics of how a disease acts in studies on the general population. Prognosis can vary depending on several factors, such as the stage of disease at diagnosis, type of disease and even gender for example cancer.

Many factors can influence the prognosis of a patient with cancer. Among the most important are the type and location of the cancer, the stage of the disease (the extent to which the cancer has spread in the body) and how quickly the cancer is likely to grow and spread. Other factors that affect prognosis include the biological and genetic properties of the cancer cells (biomarkers), the patient's age and overall general health, and the extent to which the patient's cancer responds to treatment.

Cell injury, adaptation and death

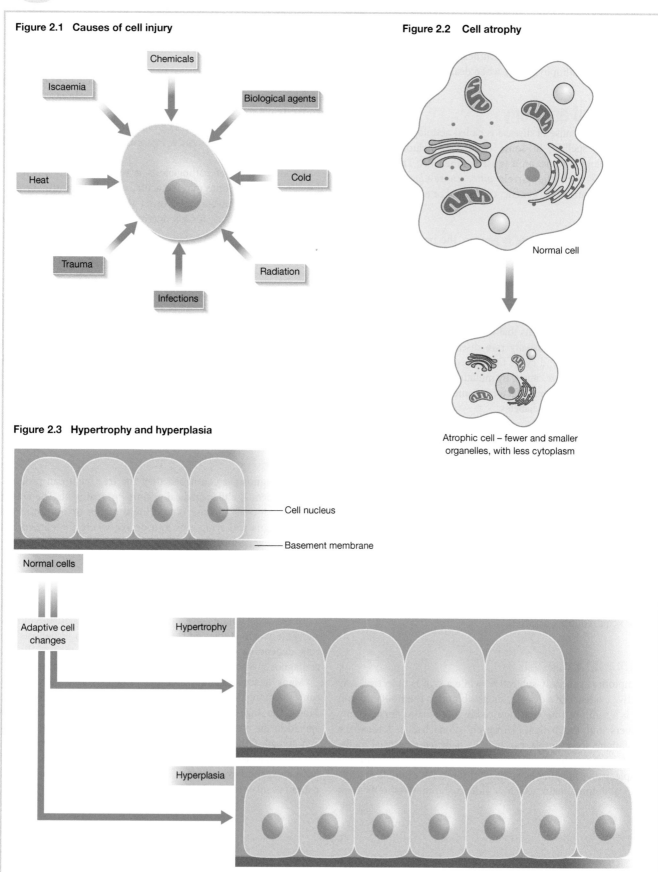

Figure 2.1   Causes of cell injury

- Chemicals
- Iscaemia
- Biological agents
- Heat
- Cold
- Trauma
- Radiation
- Infections

Figure 2.2   Cell atrophy

Normal cell

Atrophic cell – fewer and smaller organelles, with less cytoplasm

Figure 2.3   Hypertrophy and hyperplasia

- Cell nucleus
- Basement membrane

Normal cells

Adaptive cell changes

Hypertrophy

Hyperplasia

Pathophysiology for Nurses at a Glance, First Edition. Muralitharan Nair and Ian Peate. © 2015 John Wiley & Sons, Ltd. Published 2015 by John Wiley & Sons, Ltd.
Companion website: www.ataglanceseries.com/nursing/pathophysiology

Cell injury

The term 'cell injury' is used to indicate a state in which the capacity for physiological adaptation is exceeded by excessive stimuli, or when the cell is no longer capable to adapt without suffering some form of damage. Cell injury may be reversible or irreversible. Cell injury and cell death often result from exposure to toxic chemicals, infections and hypoxia (Figure 2.1).

Toxic chemicals

Chemical injury begins with the interaction between toxic chemicals and the plasma membrane. Many classes of toxic chemicals are capable of inducing acute cell injury followed by death. These include anoxia and ischaemia and their chemical analogues such as: potassium cyanide; chemical carcinogens, which form electrophiles that covalently bind to proteins in nucleic acids; oxidant chemicals, resulting in free radical formation and oxidant injury; activation of complement; and a variety of calcium ionophores. Cell death is also an important component of chemical carcinogenesis; many complete chemical carcinogens, at carcinogenic doses, produce acute necrosis and inflammation, followed by regeneration and preneoplasia.

Infections

Viruses induce cellular changes by two general mechanisms: (1) cytolytic and cytopathic viruses cause various degrees of cellular injury and cell death, (2) oncogenic viruses stimulate host cell to proliferate and may induce tumours.

Bacteria are relatively complex, single-celled creatures with a rigid wall and a thin, rubbery membrane surrounding the fluid inside the cell. They can reproduce on their own. Fossilized records show that bacteria have existed for about 3.5 billion years, and bacteria can survive in different environments, including extreme heat and cold, radioactive waste and the human body. Most bacteria are harmless, and some actually help by digesting food, destroying disease-causing microbes, fighting cancer cells and providing essential nutrients.

Hypoxia

Hypoxia is a deficiency of oxygen, which causes cell injury by reducing aerobic oxidative respiration. Hypoxia is an extremely important and common cause of cell injury and cell death. Causes of hypoxia include reduced blood flow, inadequate oxygenation of the blood due to cardiorespiratory failure and decreased oxygen-carrying capacity of the blood, as in anaemia or carbon monoxide poisoning (producing a stable carbon monoxyhaemoglobin that blocks oxygen carriage) or after severe blood loss. Depending on the severity of the hypoxic state, cells may adapt, undergo injury or die.

Adaptation

Cells adapt to the environment to escape and protect themselves from injury. Cellular adaptations are common and a central part of many disease states. The most significant adaptive states include atrophy, hypertrophy, hyperplasia and metaplasia.

Atrophy

Atrophy is a decrease or shrinkage in cell size caused by loss of subcellular organelles and substances (Figure 2.2). Atrophy can affect any , but it is most common in skeletal muscles, the heart, sex organs and the brain. However, physiological atrophy occurs in some glands. For example, the thymus gland undergoes physiological atrophy during childhood.

Hypertrophy

This is an increase in the size of the cells, thus enlarging the size of the organ (Figure 2.3). This can affect any cell but the cells of the heart, kidneys and skeletal muscles.

Hyperplasia

Hyperplasia is increased cell production in a normal tissue or organ (Figure 2.3). Hyperplasia may be a sign of abnormal or precancerous changes. This is called pathological hyperplasia. Hyperplasia may be harmless and occur on a particular tissue. An example of a normal hyperplastic response would be the growth and multiplication of milk-secreting glandular cells in the breast as a response to pregnancy, thus preparing for future breast-feeding.

Metaplasia

This is the reversible replacement of one differentiated cell type with another mature differentiated cell type. The change from one type of cell to another may generally be a part of normal maturation process or caused by some sort of abnormal stimulus. An example of metaplasia is the replacement of normal columnar ciliated epithelial cells of the bronchial lining by striated squamous epithelial cells.

Cells that die due to necrosis do not follow the apoptotic signal transduction pathway, but rather various receptors are activated that result in the loss of cell membrane integrity and an uncontrolled release of products of cell death into the intracellular space. This initiates an inflammatory response in the surrounding tissue. Nearby phagocytes are prevented from locating and engulfing the dead cells. The result is a build-up of dead tissue and cell debris at, or near, the site of the cell death.

Cell death

Cell death eventually leads to necrosis of the cell. It occurs when there is not enough blood flowing to the tissue, whether from injury, radiation, or chemicals. Necrosis is not reversible. One common type of necrosis is gangrene, which is often caused by damage from cold. There are many types of necrosis, as it can affect many areas of the body, including bone, skin, organs and other tissues.

Apoptosis

Apoptosis is derived from the Greek words *apo*, meaning away from, and *ptosis*, meaning to fall. The term 'falling away from' is derived from the fact that, during this type of prelethal change, the cells shrink and undergo marked blebbing at the periphery. The blebs then detach and float away. It is sometimes referred to as programmed cell death and, indeed, the process of apoptosis follows a controlled, predictable routine. However, it is normal for many cells to die of apoptosis as the nervous system forms; it is part of constructing appropriate connections. Apoptosis occurs in a variety of cell types following various types of toxic injury. It is especially prominent in lymphocytes, where it is the predominant mechanism for turnover of lymphocyte clones.

The resulting fragments produce the basophilic bodies seen within macrophages in lymph nodes. In other organs, apoptosis typically occurs in single cells, which are rapidly cleared away before and following death by phagocytosis of the fragments by adjacent parenchymal cells or by macrophages. Apoptosis occurring in single cells with subsequent phagocytosis typically does not result in inflammation. Prior to death, apoptotic cells show a very dense cytosol with normal or condensed mitochondria. The endoplasmic reticulum (ER) is normal or only slightly dilated.

3 Inflammation, tissue repair and regeneration

Figure 3.1 Causes of inflammation

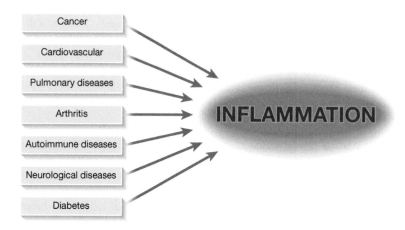

Cancer

Cardiovascular

Pulmonary diseases

Arthritis

Autoimmune diseases

Neurological diseases

Diabetes

INFLAMMATION

Figure 3.2 Tissue injury and the inflammatory process

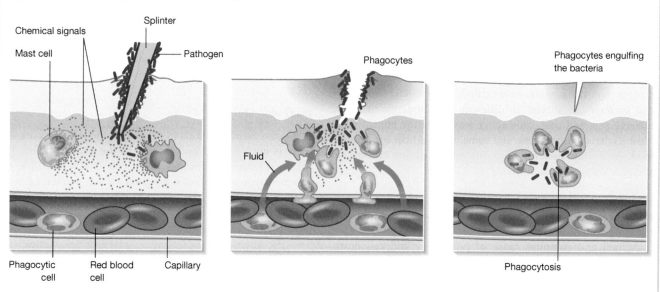

Chemical signals

Splinter

Mast cell

Pathogen

Phagocytes

Phagocytes engulfing the bacteria

Fluid

Phagocytic cell

Red blood cell

Capillary

Phagocytosis

Figure 3.3 Phases of tissue repair

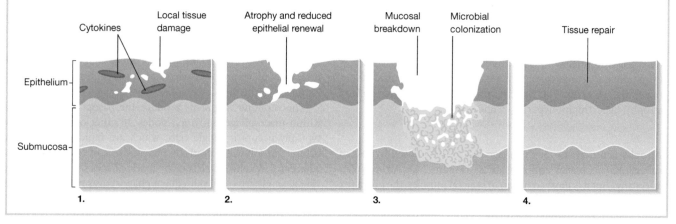

Cytokines

Local tissue damage

Atrophy and reduced epithelial renewal

Mucosal breakdown

Microbial colonization

Tissue repair

Epithelium

Submucosa

1.   2.   3.   4.

Pathophysiology for Nurses at a Glance, First Edition. Muralitharan Nair and Ian Peate. © 2015 John Wiley & Sons, Ltd. Published 2015 by John Wiley & Sons, Ltd.
Companion website: www.ataglanceseries.com/nursing/pathophysiology

Inflammation

Inflammation is the body's attempt at self-protection; the aim being to remove harmful stimuli, including damaged cells, irritants or pathogens, and begin the healing process. Inflammation can be defined clinically as the presence of swelling, redness and pain. Some diseases associated with inflammation include arthritis and neurological diseases. The signs and symptoms of inflammation are caused by four processes: (1) mast cell degranulation, (2) activation of plasma proteins, (3) the immune response and (4) heat. All these processes occur simultaneously to produce what is known as the inflammatory response. First, mast cell degranulation, is the release of granules containing serotonin and histamine from the mast cells into the tissues. These work with the other two processes below to provide the complete inflammatory signs and symptoms.

The second process involves the activation of four plasma protein systems: complement (helps to orchestrate the inflammatory response); clotting (stops bleeding and repairs damage); kinin (involved in vascular permeability); and immunoglobulins (destroy bacteria), all of which work together to support the inflammatory process. This activates and assists inflammatory and immune processes, and also plays a major role in the destruction of bacteria. The third process is the movement of phagocytic cells to the area in order to phagocytose bacteria or any other non-self debris in the wound (Figure 3.2). The fourth process, heat, is a protective attempt by the organism to remove the injurious stimuli and initiate the healing process. Without this heating, wounds would never heal.

Physical and mechanical barriers

These are part of the first-line defence against microorganisms. They include the skin and the epithelial cells of the viscera, genitourinary and respiratory tracts. The epithelial cells produce mucus to protect the lining of the tracts, some contain cilia to move the pathogens out and the temperature of the skin inhibits microorganisms from colonizing on the skin.

Biochemical barriers

Epithelial surfaces also provide both physical and biochemical barriers against infection. Some of these substances include sweat, saliva, which contains enzymes to destroy bacteria, and tears. Perspiration makes the skin pH slightly acidic, which is not a good environment for the bacteria to grow.

Acute and chronic inflammation

Acute inflammation starts rapidly (rapid onset) and quickly becomes severe. Signs and symptoms are only present for a few days, but in some cases may persist for a few weeks. Some examples include acute bronchitis, appendicitis and sore throat

Chronic inflammation means long-term inflammation, which can last for several months and even years. Some examples include chronic asthma, chronic peptic ulcer and chronic sinusitis.

Tissue repair

Wound healing, or cicatrization, is an intricate process in which the skin (or another organ-tissue) repairs itself after injury. In normal skin, the epidermis (outermost layer) and dermis (inner or deeper layer) exists in a steady-state equilibrium, forming a protective barrier against the external environment. Once the protective barrier is broken, the normal (physiological) process of wound healing is immediately set in motion. The classic model of wound healing is divided into three or four sequential, yet overlapping, phases: (1) haemostasis (not considered a phase by some), (2) inflammatory, (3) proliferative and (4) remodelling. Upon injury to the skin, a set of complex biochemical events take place in a closely orchestrated cascade to repair the damage. Within minutes post-injury, platelets (thrombocytes) aggregate at the injury site to form a fibrin clot. This clot acts to control active bleeding (haemostasis). The speed of wound healing can be impacted by many factors, including the bloodstream levels of hormones such as oxytocin.

In the inflammatory phase, bacteria and debris are phagocytosed and removed, and factors are released that cause the migration and division of cells involved in the proliferative phase.

The proliferative phase is characterized by angiogenesis, collagen deposition, granulation tissue formation, epithelialization, and wound contraction. In angiogenesis, new blood vessels are formed by vascular endothelial cells. In fibroplasia and granulation tissue formation, fibroblasts grow and form a new, provisional extracellular matrix (ECM) by excreting collagen and fibronectin. Concurrently, re-epithelialization of the epidermis occurs, in which epithelial cells proliferate and 'crawl' atop the wound bed, providing cover for the new tissue (Figure 3.3).

In contraction, the wound is made smaller by the action of myofibroblasts, which establish a grip on the wound edges and contract themselves using a mechanism similar to that in smooth muscle cells. When the cells' roles are close to complete, unneeded cells undergo apoptosis. In the maturation and remodelling phase, collagen is remodelled and realigned along tension lines and cells that are no longer needed are removed by apoptosis.

Regeneration

In the regeneration phase, blood vessels are repaired and new cells form in the damaged site, similar to the cells that were damaged and removed. Some cells, such as neurons and muscle cells (especially in the heart), are slow to recover. If the injury is minor then it is possible to return the injured tissues to their original structure and function through regeneration. However, if the injury is severe then regeneration is not possible and repair will not take place. Both regeneration and repair begin with phagocytosis, which includes fibrin from dissolved clots, microorganisms, erythrocytes and dead tissue.

Three phases occur in repairing the wound. These are the migratory, proliferative and maturation phases. In the migratory phase, the clot becomes a scab and epithelial cells migrate beneath the scab to bridge the wound. During the proliferative phase there is extensive growth of epithelial cells beneath the scab, deposition of collagen fibres by fibroblasts and continued growth of blood vessels. In the maturation phase, the scab drops off as the epidermis returns to normal thickness. In the dermis the, collagen fibres become more structured, fibroblasts decrease in number and blood vessels are restored to their normal function.

4 Cancer

Figure 4.1 Some of the organs affected by cancer

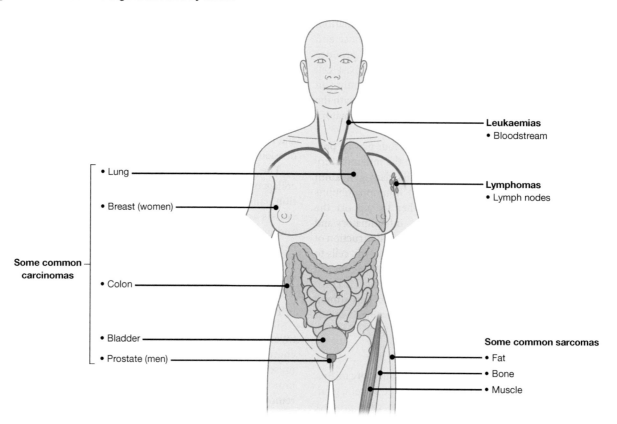

- Leukaemias
  - Bloodstream

Some common carcinomas
- Lung
- Breast (women)
- Colon
- Bladder
- Prostate (men)

- Lymphomas
  - Lymph nodes

Some common sarcomas
- Fat
- Bone
- Muscle

Figure 4.2 Staging of cancer

Different types of cancer

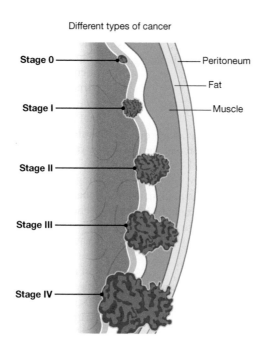

- Stage 0
- Stage I
- Stage II
- Stage III
- Stage IV

- Peritoneum
- Fat
- Muscle

What is cancer

Cancer is a disease of the cells in the body. There are many different types of cell in the body, and many different types of cancer which arise from different types of cell. What all types of cancer have in common is that the cancer cells are abnormal and multiply out of control. If not treated, the tumour can cause problems in one or more of the following ways.

Cancer can develop from almost any type of cell in the body. So there is usually more than one type of cancer that can develop in any one part of the body. Often, though, one type of cancer will be much more common in a particular organ (Figure 4.1).

For example, there are cells called transitional cells, squamous cells and adenomatous cells in the bladder. Cancer can develop in any of these cells, but is much more common in the transitional cells. Transitional cell bladder cancer is much more common than squamous cell cancer or adenocarcinoma, accounting for over nine out of ten cases of bladder cancer.

How many types of cancer are there?

It is estimated that there are more than 200 different types of cancer. Cancer can develop in any organ of the body. There are over 60 different organs in the body where a cancer can develop. Each organ is made up of several different types of cells. For example, the skin has several layers, including connective tissue, often containing gland cells. Underneath that there is often a layer of muscle tissue and so on. Each type of tissue is made up of specific types of cells.

Causes of cancer

Causes of cancers can be classified into two groups: first, there are genotoxic carcinogens which affect the DNA, causing mutations; and second, promoter substances, which may cause hormonal imbalance, altered immunity or long-term tissue damage, which can lead to the development of cancer.

Other risk factors include viruses as they weaken the immune system, hormones, such as the ones found in contraceptive pills, which can lead to breast cancer, chemical agents such as arsenic, and radiation.

Genetic factors

There need to be a number of genetic mutations within a cell before it becomes cancerous. Sometimes a person is born with one of these mutations already. This doesn't mean they will definitely get cancer. But with one mutation from the start, it makes it more likely statistically that they will develop cancer during their lifetime. Doctors call this genetic predisposition.

The BRCA1 and BRCA2 breast cancer genes are examples of genetic predisposition. Women who carry one of these faulty genes have a higher chance of developing breast cancer than women who do not.

The BRCA genes are good examples for another reason. Most women with breast cancer do not have a mutated BRCA1 or BRCA 2 gene. Less than 3% of all breast cancers are due to these genes. So although women with one of these genes are individually more likely to get breast cancer, most breast cancer is not caused by a high-risk inherited gene fault.

Age

Most types of cancer become more common as a person get older. This is because the changes that make a cell become cancerous in the first place take a long time to develop. There have to be a number of changes to the genes within a cell before it turns into a cancer cell. These changes can happen by accident when the cell is dividing, or they can happen because the cell has been damaged by carcinogens and the damage is then passed on to future cells when that cell divides. The longer a person lives the more time there is for genetic mistakes to happen in the cells.

Viruses

Viruses can help to cause some cancers. But this does not mean that these cancers can be caught like an infection. What happens is that the virus can cause genetic changes in cells that make them more likely to become cancerous.

Bacterial infection

Bacterial infections have not been thought of as cancer-causing agents in the past. But studies have shown that people who have *Helicobacter pylori* (*H pylori*) infection of their stomach develop inflammation of the stomach lining, which increases the risk of stomach cancer. *Helicobacter pylori* infection can be treated with a combination of antibiotics.

Immune system

People who have problems with their immune systems are more likely to get some types of cancer. This group includes people who have had organ transplant and HIV.

Classification/grading/staging

Diagnosis consists of naming the tumour (classification), describing its aggressiveness (grading) and reporting how far it has spread (staging). The stage of a cancer describes its size and whether it has spread beyond the area of the body where it started. The grade of a cancer depends on what the cells look like under the microscope. See Figure 4.2.

- Stage 0: is where it started (*in situ*) and not spreading.
- Stage I: the tumour is less than 2 cm and is not spreading.
- Stage II: the tumour is 2–5 cm with or without lymph node involvement (lymph nodes are part of the lymphatic system). It has not spread.
- Stage III: the tumour is more than 5 cm, or any size, but fixed either to the chest wall, muscle or skin, or has spread to lymph nodes above the collarbone.
- Stage IV: the tumour is any size – it may affect the lymph nodes but has definitely spread to other parts of the body.

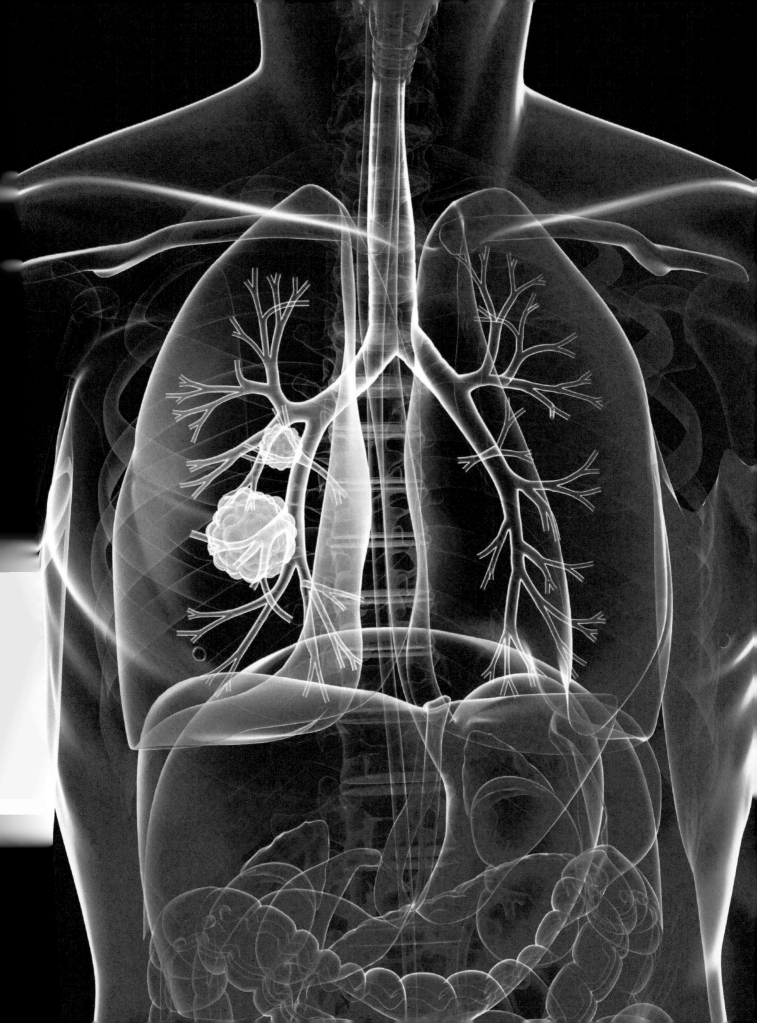

Anaphylaxis is a serious, potentially life-threatening allergic response that is marked by swelling, hives, hypotension and dilated blood vessels. In severe cases shock may occur and if anaphylactic shock is not treated immediately, it can result in death.

Anaphylaxis occurs when the immune system develops a specific antibody (called immunoglobulin E, or IgE) that drives an inappropriate or exaggerated reaction toward a substance that is usually harmless, for example food. The body may not react upon initial exposure but may produce antibodies with later exposures. When exposed to the substance later, the binding of the allergen to antibodies can lead to the presence of a large amount of histamine (a protein) being produced, causing the symptoms identified above.

Anaphylactic shock

Anaphylaxis can occur within seconds or minutes of exposure to something the person is allergic to, for example the venom from a bee sting. The immune system releases a flood of chemicals during anaphylaxis that can cause shock. Common triggers of anaphylaxis include certain foods, some medications, insect venom and latex. Anaphylaxis requires immediate emergency treatment; if the condition is not treated right away, unconsciousness or even death can occur. See Figure 6.1.

Pathophysiology

The number of those who suffer severe systemic allergic reactions is growing; however, as anaphylaxis is not always recognized, the incidence may be under-reported.

An anaphylactic reaction happens when an allergen reacts with specific IgE antibodies on mast cells and basophils (type 1 hypersensitivity reaction). This triggers the rapid release of stored histamine and the rapid synthesis of newly formed mediators. As a result these cause capillary leakage, mucosal oedema and eventually shock and asphyxia. Anaphylactic reactions can vary in severity and rate of progression; they may progress rapidly (over a few minutes) or sometimes in a biphasic manner. Rarely, manifestations may be delayed by a few hours (this adds to diagnostic difficulty), or continue for more than 24 hours. Anaphylactoid reactions are not IgE-mediated but cause similar mast cell activation. A significant number of cases of anaphylaxis are idiopathic. Table 6.1 identifies the most common triggers of anaphylaxis.

Signs and symptoms

There is usually (but not always) a previous history of sensitivity to an allergen, or recent history of exposure to a new drug. Primarily, people often develop skin symptoms, including generalized itching, urticaria and erythema, rhinitis, conjunctivitis and angio-oedema. If the airway is becoming involved signs may include itching of the palate or external auditory meatus, dyspnoea, stridor (laryngeal oedema) and bronchospasm. General symptoms comprise palpitations and tachycardia, nausea, vomiting and abdominal pain, a fainting feeling, with a sense of impending doom; ultimately the person will collapse and lose consciousness. If there is airway swelling, stridor, dysnpoea, bronchospasm, cyanosis, hypotension, tachycardia and reduced capillary filling then these are suggestive of an approaching severe reaction.

Investigations

Anaphylaxis is diagnosed based on its symptoms. Those with a history of allergic reactions may be at greater risk for developing a severe reaction in the future. Skin testing can help confirm the substances that cause severe allergic reactions. However, this type of test may not be recommended if there is a reason to suspect that the person will have an anaphylactic reaction to the substance.

Serum mast-cell tryptase can be measured in order to clarify diagnosis where ambiguity exists. Tryptase is the preferred marker demonstrating mast-cell degranulation. Levels of serum tryptase, which is a mast-cell specific protease, are highest at one hour post an anaphylactic reaction, staying elevated for about six hours. Elevated serum tryptase levels imply massive mast-cell degranulation (occurring in anaphylaxis) or a condition such as mastocytosis. Not all cases of anaphylaxis result in a rise in tryptase.

National guidance exists concerning the identification and management of anaphylaxis. The essential principles of treatment are the same for all age groups.

Diagnosis of anaphylaxis is a clinical one, beginning with a brief, directed history, as treatment must be provided quickly. This history includes questions about a previous history of atopy or anaphylaxis and exposure to new foods, medications and insect bites or stings.

Management

Rapid assessment:

Airway: look for and relieve airway obstruction; call for help early if there are signs of obstruction. Remove any traces of allergen remaining (e.g. nut fragments caught in teeth, with a mouthwash, bee stings, without compressing any attached venom sacs).

Breathing: look for and treat bronchospasm and signs of respiratory distress.

Circulation: colour, pulse and BP.

Disability: assess whether responding or unconscious.

Exposure: assess skin with adequate exposure, but avoid excess heat loss.

High-flow oxygen is given using a mask with an oxygen reservoir (greater than 10 litres per minute to prevent reservoir collapse). The person is placed flat: Epinephrine injection is the only rapidly effective treatment for anaphylaxis; epinephrine rapidly reverses anaphylactic symptoms. It is typically given through an automatic injection device. The most common and most effective injection site is the thigh. Large-bore intravenous cannulae are inserted and a rapid fluid challenge is administered. Assessment of central venous pressure is required. Chlorphenamine and hydrocortisone are given after initial resuscitation. Pulse oximetry, electrocardiograph and blood pressure are monitored.

Those patients prone to anaphylaxis should be provided with one or more auto-injector kits and should be instructed on their use. The patient should be advised to carry the auto-injector kit on their person at all times.

7 Hypovolaemic shock

Figure 7.1 Sequence of events in hypovolaemic shock

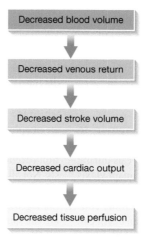

Decreased blood volume

↓

Decreased venous return

↓

Decreased stroke volume

↓

Decreased cardiac output

↓

Decreased tissue perfusion

Table 7.1 Stages of hypovolaemic shock

Compensated shock	Baroreceptor reflexes result in increase in myocardial contractility, tachycardia and vasoconstriction. They maintain cardiac output and BP and lead to the release of vasopressin, aldosterone and renin
Progressive or uncompensated shock	Occurs with myocardial depression, failure of vasomotor reflexes and failure of the microcirculation, with increase in capillary permeability, sludging and thrombosis, resulting in cellular dysfunction and lactic acidosis
Irreversible shock	Failure of vital organs, with inability to recover

Table 7.2 The fundamentals of management

General measures	• Oxygen should be given • Venous access is required early • Resuscitation usually begins with crystalloid, such as normal saline or Hartmann's solution. Albumin may play a role in those requiring substantial amounts of crystalloid to maintain a mean arterial pressure in the setting of septic shock. In haemorrhage, blood should be given as soon as possible • A central venous pressure line may be required
Pharmacological	• Vasodilator therapy may be required. It is used more for septic shock. If hypovolaemia occurs then circulating blood volume should be increased • Analgesia must be given by the intravenous route; any other route will be ineffective. Pain increases metabolic rate and so aggravates tissue ischaemia
Surgical	• Surgery may be needed if bleeding continues to stem the flow. It is normal to resuscitate first, reducing the risk, as induction of anaesthesia can lead to collapse of a fragile circulation • In trauma, first aid measures may help stem blood loss. In gunshot wounds look for not just the entrance but also the exit wound. The latter may be significantly larger than the former. If a high-powered weapon was used, primary closure of the wound should not be attempted

Pathophysiology for Nurses at a Glance, First Edition. Muralitharan Nair and Ian Peate. © 2015 John Wiley & Sons, Ltd. Published 2015 by John Wiley & Sons, Ltd.
Companion website: www.ataglanceseries.com/nursing/pathophysiology

Hypovolaemic shock occurs when the volume in the circulatory system is too depleted to allow adequate circulation to vital organs and tissues of the body. Resuscitation aims to correct the hypovolaemia and hypoperfusion of vital organs, such as the brain and kidneys, prior to irreversible damage occurring.

Hypovolaemic shock

Hypovolaemic shock is a medical or surgical condition; rapid fluid loss results in multiple organ failure as a result of inadequate circulating volume, causing inadequate perfusion. Hypovolaemic shock is very often due to rapid blood loss (sometimes referred to as haemorrhagic shock).

Two common causes of haemorrhagic shock are acute, external blood loss secondary to penetrating trauma and severe gastrointestinal bleeding. It can also be caused by a significant acute internal bleed into the thoracic and abdominal cavities. Hypovolaemic shock can result from significant fluid loss, other than blood loss, for example fluid loss due to severe gastroenteritis and extensive burns.

Pathophysiology

Without fluid and blood resuscitation and/or correction of the underlying pathology causing the haemorrhage, cardiac perfusion eventually diminishes, and multiple organ failure soon follows.

There are a number of causes of hypovolaemic shock, including loss of blood; this can be revealed or occult. Trauma can lead to visible bleeding or rupture of an internal organ such as the spleen or liver. A fractured femur can bleed approximately half a litre and a fractured pelvis will lose about one litre of blood (note these volumes vary according to age/weight). The amount of haematemesis indicates the degree of bleeding. Bleeding as a result of ectopic pregnancy is also occult, with little or no vaginal loss. Blood loss and leakage of plasma occurs in burns. Severe loss of water and salt occurs with strenuous exercise in a hot environment, poor fluid intake, loss from diarrhoea and vomiting, and inappropriate diuresis. Other causes of shock include, poor cardiac output as is the case in massive myocardial infarction, ruptured aortic valve or massive pulmonary embolism, septic shock and acute pancreatitis, leading to a fall in vascular resistance and high transection of the spine or a high spinal anaesthetic.

A healthy adult can endure the loss of half a litre from a circulation of approximately five litres without adverse effect; larger volumes and rapid loss, however, result in progressively greater problems. Risk is related to the degree of hypovolaemia as well as the speed of correction. The risk of morbidity and mortality grows as age increases. Unfavorable pathology in the cardiovascular, respiratory and renal systems can increase risk.

The human body has an ability to respond to acute haemorrhage by activating the following major physiological systems: the haematological, cardiovascular, renal and neuroendocrine systems. The haematological system responds to a severe acute blood loss by triggering the coagulation cascade and contracting the bleeding vessels (releasing local thromboxane A_2 release). Platelets are activated and form an immature clot on the source of bleeding. The damaged vessel exposes collagen; this subsequently causes fibrin deposition and stabilization of the clot.

Initially the cardiovascular system responds to hypovolaemic shock by increasing the heart rate, increasing myocardial contractility and constricting peripheral blood vessels. This occurs secondary to an increased release of norepinephrine and decreased baseline vagal tone (the baroreceptors in the carotid arch, aortic arch, left atrium and pulmonary vessels regulate this). The cardiovascular system redistributes blood to the brain, heart and kidneys and away from skin, muscle and gastrointestinal tract.

The renal system responds to haemorrhagic shock, stimulating an increase in the secretion of renin from the juxtaglomerular apparatus. Angiotensinogen is converted to angiotensin I by renin, which is then converted to angiotensin II by the lungs and liver. Angiotensin II has two important effects, both of these help to reverse haemorrhagic shock, vasoconstriction of arteriolar smooth muscle and stimulation of aldosterone secretion by the adrenal cortex.

The neuroendocrine system responds to haemorrhagic shock by causing an increase in circulating antidiuretic hormone (ADH). This is released from the posterior pituitary gland in response to a decrease in blood pressure (detected by baroreceprors) and a decrease in the sodium concentration (detected by osmoreceptors). ADH indirectly leads to an increased reabsorption of water and sodium chloride by the distal tubule, the collecting ducts, and the loop of Henle.

The pathophysiology of hypovolaemic shock is complex; there are many intricate mechanisms that are effective in maintaining vital organ perfusion in severe blood loss. See Figure 7.1.

Signs and symptoms

The person might feel cold, unwell, anxious, faint and short of breath. There may be faintness on standing or even on sitting up, related to postural hypotension. There may be symptoms related to the cause of the hypovolaemia, for example as pain from a haemorrhaging ulcer, dissecting aneurysm, ruptured ectopic pregnancy, trauma or burns. Nausea and vomiting can be related to gut ischaemia. The patient may look pale and sweaty, with tachypnoea. The periphery may be cold due to poor perfusion; capillary refill time may be prolonged. There may be tachycardia and hypotension or postural hypotension. Tachycardia is often a later feature than the cold periphery, and hypotension occurs still later. Late features include confusion or even coma. Physiologically there are three stages of hypovolaemic shock (Table 7.1).

Investigations

These include full blood count, urea and electrolytes, liver function tests, coagulation screen and arterial blood gas analysis. Ultrasound is used for differentiating hypovolaemic from cardiogenic shock; the vena cava can be assessed for adequate filling. Echocardiogram may demonstrate pump failure. Central venous pressure monitoring may be of value where there is evidence of shock.

Management

Rapid volume repletion is required in those with hypovolaemic shock. Delayed therapy can lead to ischaemic injury and potentially to irreversible shock and multi-organ system failure. Table 7.2 outlines the fundamentals of management.

8 Septicaemia

Table 8.1 Sepsis: a disease continuum

Group	Description
Systemic inflammatory response syndrome (SIRS)	This is a clinical response arising from a non-specific insult and including 2 or more of the following: • Temperature above 38°C or less than 36°C; heart rate above 90 beats per minute • Respiratory rate lest than 20 per minute with abnormal arterial blood gas results • A raised white blood cell count
Sepsis	As above with apparent or confirmed infectious process
Severe sepsis	Sepsis with one or more signs of: • Organ dysfunction • Poor perfusion (hypoperfusion) • Hypotension • Oliguria • Respiratory failure • Confusion or altered mental state

Table 8.2 Some risk factors associated with the development of sepsis

• Those who are elderly and those who are very young

• Instrumentation or surgery

• Alcohol abuse

• People with diabetes mellitus

• Those with burns

• Immunosuppression

• Those who have undergone organ transplantation

• People who are undernourished

• Certain medications, such as high dose steroids, chemotherapy

Table 8.3 The mnemonic SEPSIS

Slurred speech
Extreme muscle pain
Passing no urine
Severe breathlessness
I feel I might die
Skin mottled or discoloured

Table 8.4 The six interventions for septic shock as outlined by the UK Sepsis Trust

1. Provision of high flow oxygen therapy
2. Taking blood cultures
3. Administration of broad spectrum antibiotics
4. Provision of intravenous fluid
5. Measurement of serum lactate and haemoglobin
6. Measurement of hourly urine output

Pathophysiology for Nurses at a Glance, First Edition. Muralitharan Nair and Ian Peate. © 2015 John Wiley & Sons, Ltd. Published 2015 by John Wiley & Sons, Ltd.
Companion website: www.ataglanceseries.com/nursing/pathophysiology

Sepsis remains a serious problem, bringing with it substantial morbidity and mortality. It is a serious clinical problem accounting for thousands of deaths annually.

When discussing septic shock there are a variety of terms and definitions used. Whilst many of them are similar, there are differences. Sepsis and septicemia refer to a number of ill-defined clinical conditions present in a patient with bacteraemia. In clinical practice these terms are often used interchangeably.

Bacteraemia means that there is the presence of bacteria in the blood. Usually when there is only a small amount of bacteria this is dealt with by the person's immune system and as a result there are no systemic effects. When more bacteria are present this can cause systemic signs and symptoms with a number of sequelae, such as pneumonia or abscess formation; this can be with or without sepsis. Septicaemia occurs when there is the presence of abundant bacteria in the blood and they are vigorously dividing. This causes a systemic response that leads to organ dysfunction. Septicaemia is a critical illness and can be fatal; this can be complicated by a number of life-threatening conditions, for example circulatory collapse. This condition is serious and should never be considered as just an infection.

Pathophysiology

Sepsis should be considered as a disease continuum (see Table 8.1). The pathophysiology associated with septic shock is not exactly understood; however, it involves a multifaceted interaction between the pathogen and the individual's immune system. The usual physiological reaction to a localized infection will include the initiation of host defence mechanisms, causing an increase of white blood cells, along with the release of inflammatory mediators, local vasodilation, increased leakage of fluid from blood vessels and the initiation of the various blood clotting pathways. Sepsis entails a variety of disorders, for example abnormal coagulation, damage to the blood vessel lining, presence of tumour necrosis factor in excessive amounts and deficiency of steroid hormones.

There are a variety of causes of septic shock and bacterial infection is most common; generally this is responsive to antibiotic therapy. Sometimes the infection can overwhelm the person's defence mechanisms and progress rapidly to a serious illness called severe sepsis.

Pneumonia, perforated bowel, urinary tract infection and severe skin infections are the most frequent causes of severe sepsis. Infections as a result of childbirth are not common, but overall this is the foremost cause of direct maternal death. There is usually an abscess or a nidus (a focus) of infection associated with sepsis. Some risk factors for developing sepsis are outlined in Table 8.2.

Signs and symptoms

Sepsis is the existence (probable or documented) of infection, along with systemic signs of infection. Severe sepsis, however, is described as sepsis with sepsis-induced organ dysfunction or tissue hypoperfusion. In order to help you remember the signs and symptoms of sepsis the mnemonic SEPSIS may help (see Table 8.3).

The person may have been to see the practice nurse or GP and presented a few days earlier with a focus of infection. Antibiotics may have been prescribed for the condition. However, despite this their condition may have declined quickly. Often the person presents with symptoms that are non-specific, such as, tiredness, nausea and vomiting, abdominal pain and diarrhoea. The person may appear unwell, and there may be a spiking temperature that may or may not be accompanied by rigors. Tachycardia may be present, with a bounding pulse. There may be tachypnoea, along with cyanosis. The individual may have cold peripheries (they feel cold to touch) and they may also be sweating. Hypotension may be present. Drowsiness and impaired consciousness can occur; in the older person this is common. Other features will relate to the infection itself, there may be a rash, the signs of a wound infection, the person may be wheezing or chest crackles can be heard in pneumonia. The nurse needs to understand that the features outlined here may not be present in the elderly. In those people who are immunocompromised these features may not be present.

Investigations

It is usual for a diagnosis to be made based on the clinical features the person presents with. A full blood count will be required, determining the presence of anaemia or other blood disorders; urinary tract infection needs to be ruled out. Renal function tests help to determine if there is dehydration or organ failure. Liver function tests can help to assess if there is liver damage. Blood cultures will be required. A chest X-ray, abdominal ultrasound and CT scan are needed. Oxygen saturation levels and an analysis of arterial blood gases are required. Invasive investigations may be required if the infection is covert, such as, lumbar puncture or bronchoscopy.

Management

Those with septic shock are transferred to the intensive care unit, receiving ongoing support for organ dysfunction. The majority of patients require mechanical ventilation and treatment to support cardiac function. If renal impairment is present haemofiltration may be needed, with haematological support for problems associated with abnormal blood clotting.

In preventing progression from infection and sepsis to death (the sepsis continuum) practitioners must have skills that can help identify key clinical indicators; timely and appropriate interventions are required in order to prevent complications and to avoid death.

The six interventions for septic shock outlined by the UK Sepsis Trust are detailed in Table 8.4. These six interventions must be carried out within an hour.

In an appropriate care environment, such as intensive care unit, supportive care will include the need to resuscitate the person. Intravenous rehydration will be required; intravenous hydrocortisone may be administered, along with fludrocortisone. Monitoring the person's condition will be required, for example pulse, temperature, respiratory rate, rhythm and depth, blood pressure, oxygen saturation, central venous pressure and also hourly urinary output.

Broad spectrum intravenous antibiotics are given in the first instance. Unusual organisms, including fungi, will require specific treatment with specialist input from a microbiologist and virologist.

Surgery may be needed to debride wounds or drain an abscess.

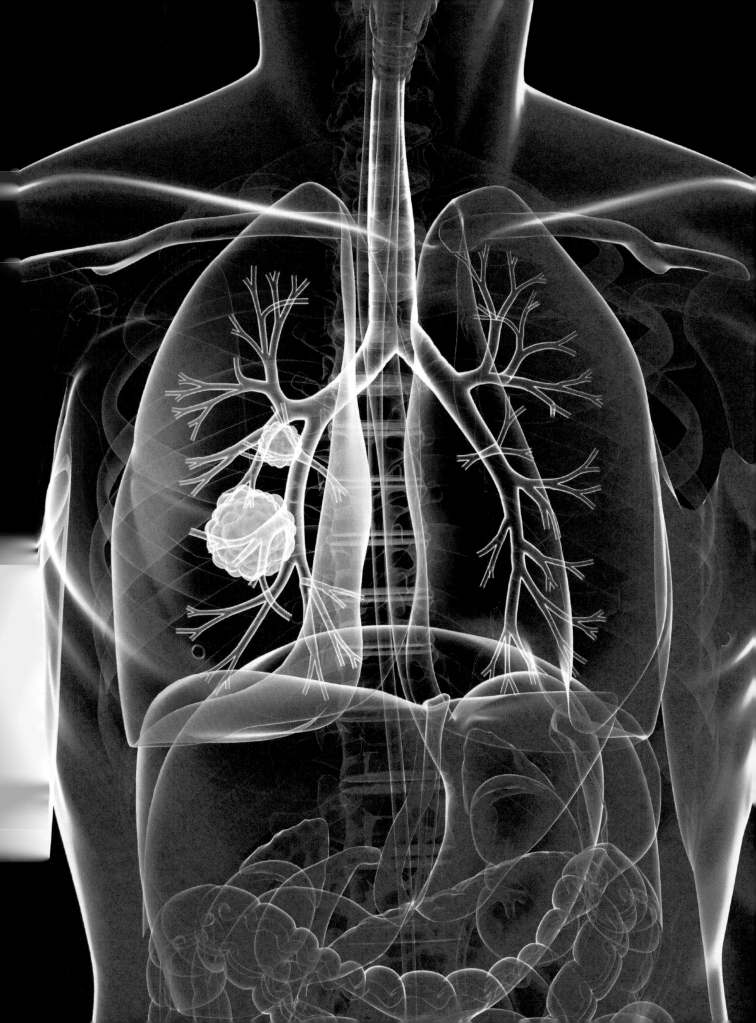

Non-Hodgkin lymphoma

Non-Hodgkin lymphomas (NHLs) are the fifth most common cancer in the UK, with approximately 11,500 people diagnosed with it annually. There are several different types of NHL. Some of them will grow very slowly and treatment may not be required for months or years: other types have a tendency to grow quickly and treatment is required soon after a diagnosis is made. Non-Hodgkin's lymphoma is associated with ageing. As a person ages there are increased chances of developing the condition. At diagnosis the average age is around 65. Risk is higher in white people than black and Asian people.

Pathophysiology

Non-Hodgkin lymphomas (NHLs) are a heterogeneous group of tumours that originate from lymphoid tissues, primarily of lymph nodes (a type of cancer of the lymphatic system) (see Figures 10.1 and 10.2.) They are lymphoproliferative malignancies with differing patterns of behaviour and responses to treatment; the prognosis depends on the histological type, stage and treatment. With NHLs there is a much greater tendency for the malignancy to disseminate to extranodal sites than is the case with Hodgkin's lymphoma.

NHL is associated with an altered or defective immune system; the incidence of the illness is higher in those people who are receiving immunosuppressive medications for organ transplant, people with HIV and those people with certain viral conditions, for example Epstein-Barr virus. Some risk factors include having a family member with the condition (family history), being male, being white, having an autoimmune disease such as rheumatoid arthritis and having been exposed to radiotherapy.

NHL may result from chromosomal translocations, infections, environmental factors, immunodeficiency states and chronic inflammation. The malignant biochemical characteristic in NHL is due to abnormal gene mutations occurring during lymphocyte production, maturation or action. The transformations lead to growth advantage and expansion of a monoclonal population of malignant lymphocytes. The type of lymphoma (B cell or T cell) depends on the stage of lymphocyte production, maturation or action at which mutation occurs.

B-cell lymphoma

The process of B-cell production is still undergoing much research. It is thought that B cells originate and mature in the bone marrow (the central lymphoid tissue compartment). They may leave bone marrow to perform their function in lymph nodes and extranodal tissues (e.g. peripheral lymphoid tissue compartment).

The abnormal mutations can occur at the stage of early precursors, leading to corresponding subtypes of acute lymphoblastic leukaemia. Immature B cells, mature antigen-naive B cells and mature antigen-activated B cells may transform to various types of NHL, such as Burkitt's lymphoma, diffuse large B-cell lymphoma and mantle cell lymphoma.

T-cell lymphoma

The exact cause of most T-cell lymphomas is unknown. However, it is likely that genetic changes that take place during antigen processing and presentation result in an aggressively dividing cell population that may give rise to T-cell lymphoma. In contrast to B cells, T cells migrate early into the thymus, where they develop into mature cells. The abnormal mutations can happen at different stages of T-cell development and can lead to different malignant phenotypes.

Signs and symptoms

The clinical manifestations vary with such factors as the location of the lymphomatous process, speed of tumour growth and the function of the organ compromised or displaced by the malignancy. Clinical manifestations can include:

Low-grade lymphomas:
- Painless, slowly progressive, peripheral lymphadenopathy
- Primary extranodal involvement
- Fatigue, weakness, fever, night sweats, weight loss
- Cytopenia
- Splenomegaly
- Hepatomegaly

Intermediate and high-grade lymphomas:
- Rapidly growing, bulky lymphadenopathy
- Systemic symptoms and extranodal involvement
- Hepatomegaly
- Splenomegaly
- Testicular mass
- Skin lesions: associated with cutaneous T-cell lymphoma
- Burkitt's lymphoma: presents with a large abdominal mass and symptoms of bowel obstruction
- Pulmonary involvement, superior vena obstruction

Investigations

- Full blood count
- Renal function tests and electrolytes
- Serology: HIV, HTLV-1, hepatitis C
- Chest X-ray
- Lymph node excision core biopsy is for the diagnosis of follicular lymphoma; histology for assessment of the tumour grade
- CT scan of neck, chest, abdomen and pelvis
- Bone scans
- Whole body positron emission tomography (PET) scan
- Scrotal ultrasound
- Lumbar puncture

Other investigations may be indicated, depending on the clinical presentation.

Management

Treatment options vary because of the mixed nature of NHLs: the type and grade of NHL, stage of NHL and the person's general health. Options include watchful waiting, single-agent or multi-agent chemotherapy and regional or extended radiotherapy. Surgery in treatment is limited but may be useful in certain situations. Those with severe neutropenia should be given antibiotic prophylaxis with chemotherapy. Monoclonal antibodies (rituximab, a biological therapy) may be given with chemotherapy.

11 Infectious mononucleosis

Figure 11.1   Lymphadenopathy

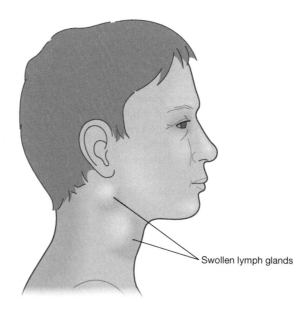

Swollen lymph glands

Figure 11.2   The main symptoms of infectious mononucleosis

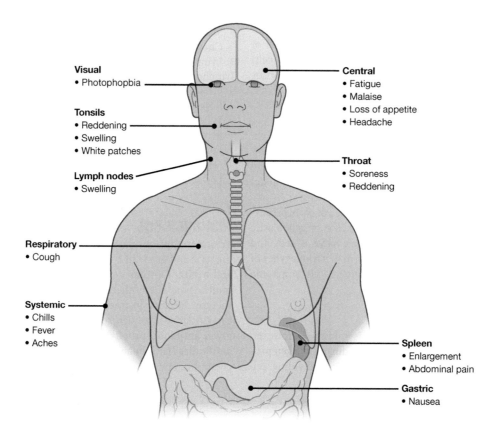

Visual
• Photophopbia

Tonsils
• Reddening
• Swelling
• White patches

Lymph nodes
• Swelling

Respiratory
• Cough

Systemic
• Chills
• Fever
• Aches

Central
• Fatigue
• Malaise
• Loss of appetite
• Headache

Throat
• Soreness
• Reddening

Spleen
• Enlargement
• Abdominal pain

Gastric
• Nausea

Pathophysiology for Nurses at a Glance, First Edition. Muralitharan Nair and Ian Peate. © 2015 John Wiley & Sons, Ltd. Published 2015 by John Wiley & Sons, Ltd.
Companion website: www.ataglanceseries.com/nursing/pathophysiology

Infectious mononucleosis is also known as glandular fever.

Infectious mononucleosis

Infectious mononucleosis is a clinical syndrome that consists of fever, pharyngitis and adenopathy (enlargement or swelling of the lymph nodes). Most cases of glandular fever are caused by the Epstein-Barr virus (EBV) which is one of the most common viruses to affect humans. It is a member of the herpes virus family.

EBV is a viral infection that predominately affects younger adults. The majority of adults show evidence of previous EBV infection in analysis of blood (serology). It is not usually a serious threat to a person's health, but glandular fever can be unpleasant and may last several weeks. If a person develops an EBV infection during early adulthood, they can develop symptoms of glandular fever.

Pathophysiology

The EBV is transmitted via intimate contact with body secretions, primarily oropharyngeal secretions. EBV can be spread through kissing (it is sometimes referred to as the 'kissing disease'), exposure to coughs and sneezes, sharing of eating and drinking utensils, for example cups, glasses and unwashed forks and spoons.

EBV infects the B cells in the epithelium of the oropharynx. There are some instances where genital transmission can occur where the organism may also be shed from the uterine cervix. Rarely, EBV can be transmitted via blood transfusion.

Circulating B cells spread the infection throughout the entire reticular endothelial system, that is, the liver, spleen and the peripheral lymph nodes. EBV infection of B lymphocytes causes a humoral and cellular response to the virus. The humoral immune response directed against the EBV structural proteins is the basis for the test that is used to diagnose EBV infectious mononucleosis. The T-lymphocyte response, however, is essential in the control of EBV infection; natural killer cells and principally CD8+ cytotoxic T cells control growing B lymphocytes that have been infected with EBV.

The T-lymphocyte cellular response is significant in influencing the clinical expression of EBV viral infection. A rapid and efficient T-cell response results in control of the primary EBV infection as well as lifelong suppression of EBV.

T-cell response that is ineffective can lead to excessive and uncontrolled B-cell proliferation, resulting in B-lymphocyte malignancies (e.g. B-cell lymphomas).

Fever is the immune response to EBV infection and this occurs because of cytokine release as a result of B-lymphocyte invasion by EBV. Lymphocytosis seen in the reticular endothelial system is caused by the multiplication of EBV-infected B lymphocytes. Pharyngitis in EBV infectious mononucleosis is caused by the proliferation of EBV-infected B lymphocytes in the lymphatic tissue of the oropharynx (see Figure 11.1).

Signs and symptoms

The majority of people infected with EBV are asymptomatic. The incubation period (the time from infection to appearance of symptoms) ranges from four to six weeks. People with infectious mononucleosis can transmit the infection to others for a period of weeks. Once a person has had glandular fever, it is highly unlikely they will develop a second infection as most people develop a lifelong immunity to glandular fever after the primary infection.

The majority of people with infectious mononucleosis complain of fatigue and prolonged malaise. A sore throat is second only to fatigue and malaise as a presenting symptom. A low grade pyrexia is often present. Arthralgia and myalgia can occur; however, these are less common than in other viral infectious diseases. Nausea and anorexia, without vomiting, are common symptoms.

A number of other symptoms have been described in people with infectious mononucleosis, for example cough, ocular muscle pain, chest pain and photophobia. Splenomegaly may occur. See Figure 11.2.

Investigations

Infection with EBV provokes specific antibodies to EBV and also various unrelated non-EBV heterophile antibodies (antibodies against an antigen produced in one species that react against antigens from other species). These heterophile antibodies are not specific for the virus.

As the symptoms caused by infectious mononucleosis are similar to symptoms that are due to a number of other viruses it can be difficult to diagnose infectious mononucleosis by clinical examination alone. Blood tests are carried out in order to detect antibodies and confirm the diagnosis of glandular fever. These antibodies can be detected by a Paul-Bunnell test and Monospot® test.

Positivity increases during the first six weeks of the illness and so the heterophile antibody test results may be negative early in the course of infectious mononucleosis and, as such, blood tests may need to be repeated.

Management

If there is evidence or a suspicion of splenic involvement patients are advised to avoid contact sports for three weeks, as there may be a risk of splenic rupture. Paracetamol should be given for its analgesic and antipyretic properties. There is no specific antiviral therapy available. If there is extreme tonsillar enlargement then a short course of corticosteroids may be beneficial. In uncomplicated infectious mononucleosis there is no specific treatment; interventions should aim to enhance comfort. The person should be encouraged to drink plenty of fluids.

In order to prevent onwards transmission, kissing and close body contact with other people should be avoided. The person should be advised not to share cups, towels, etc. Alcohol should be avoided.

It is anticipated that a person will make a full recovery usually within 14 days. However, malaise, tiredness, myalgia and arthralgia can last a few weeks or even months longer.

Admission to hospital to correct dehydration and to provide fluid replacement may be required.

Potential complications

- Extreme tonsillar enlargement can cause upper airway obstruction
- Myocarditis and cardiac conduction abnormalities
- Splenic rupture
- Haemolytic anaemia, thrombocytopenia
- Acute interstitial nephritis, glomerulonephritis
- Neurological, including aseptic meningitis, encephalitis, cranial nerve palsies or Guillain-Barré syndrome
- Prolonged fatigue; depression

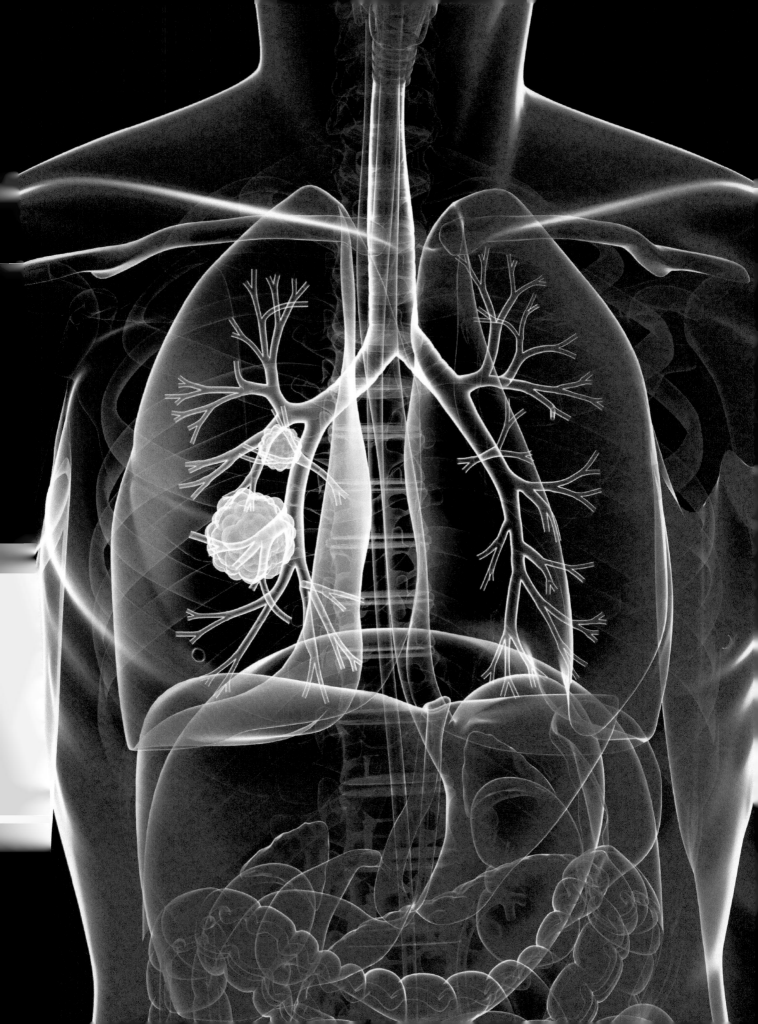

Overview of anatomy and physiology

MS is a disease affecting nerves in the brain and spinal cord, causing problems with muscle movement, balance and vision. Each nerve fibre in the brain and spinal cord is surrounded by a layer of protein called myelin (Figure 13.1), which protects the nerve and helps electrical signals from the brain travel to the rest of the body.

Many thousands of nerve fibres transmit tiny electrical impulses (messages) between different parts of the brain and spinal cord. Each nerve fibre in the brain and spinal cord is surrounded by a protective sheath made from a substance called myelin. The myelin sheath acts like the insulation around an electrical wire, and is needed for the electrical impulses to travel correctly along the nerve fibre (Figure 13.2). In MS, the myelin becomes damaged.

Pathophysiology

MS is thought to be an autoimmune disease. This means that cells of the immune system, which normally attack bacteria and viruses, attack part of the body. When the disease is active, parts of the immune system, mainly cells called T cells, attack the myelin sheath which surrounds the nerve fibres in the brain and spinal cord. This leads to small patches of inflammation.

The inflammation around the myelin sheath stops the affected nerve fibres from working properly, and symptoms develop. When the inflammation clears, the myelin sheath may heal and repair, and nerve fibres start to work again. However, the inflammation, or repeated bouts of inflammation, can leave a small scar (sclerosis), which can permanently damage nerve fibres. In a typical person with MS, many (multiple) small areas of scarring (sclerosis) develop in the brain and spinal cord. These scars may also be called plaques.

The inflammation destroys myelin and oligodendrocytes, in patches called plaques along the axon, leading to axon dysfunction. The demyelination (Figure 13.3) and plaque formation results in scarring of the glia and degeneration of the axons.

Signs and symptoms

MS causes a wide variety of symptoms. Many people experience only a few symptoms and it is very unlikely that a person will develop all the symptoms described here. Symptoms of MS are usually unpredictable.

Some people find that their symptoms worsen gradually with time. More commonly, symptoms come and go at different times. Periods when symptoms worsen are called relapses. Periods when symptoms improve (or even disappear altogether) are called remissions.

Relapses can occur at any time and symptoms may differ within each relapse. Although relapses usually occur for no apparent reason, various triggers can include infections, exercise and even hot weather. The symptoms that occur during a relapse depend on which part, or parts, of the brain or spinal cord are affected. Patients may have just one symptom in one part of the body, or several symptoms in different parts of the body. The symptoms occur because the affected nerve fibres stop working properly.

Diagnosis

Diagnosis for MS is challenging because the disease does not present uniformly and there is no single test to confirm diagnosis. MS is diagnosed through historical assessment of the patient, neurological assessments, MRI scans of the brain, CSF analysis through lumbar puncture and evoked response testing (visual, auditory, somatosensory), which may show delayed nerve conduction.

Management

Many people with MS learn to lead a normal life at home, requiring hospital admission when the disease is getting worse and they have complications such as a chest infection or inability to cope. Hospital admission during the advancement of the disease process may cause severe stress, especially for the person whose daily routine is disrupted as a result of the hospital admission.

The disease process affects young adults in their prime of life. The psychological and economical effect can be devastating for the patient and their relatives. People with MS will have to make adjustments to their body image changes and at the same time learn to cope with the disease. The unpredicatable course of the disease is a challenging situation for any healthcare provider.

Interventions for the person with MS vary with the coping strategies of the person and their relatives. Many of the nursing interventions relate to the inability of the person to perform activities of daily living.

The person with MS will complain of fatigue with or without exertion. Fatigue affects every aspect of the life of the person with MS. Nurses can help the person and their family to understand how to prevent fatigue and exacerbations. The daily activities should include rest periods and psychological relaxation. Encourage the person with MS to avoid extreme temperatures (hot or cold) as they can delay transmission of impulses across demyelinated neurones, which contributes to fatigue.

Maintaining mobility plays a large part in being independent. The person with MS may need assistance, depending on the advancement of the disease, in undertaking short walks. Healthcare providers should work as a team to encourage a positive outlook for the patient, while taking time to understand the patients and their relatives' fears and feelings.

The person with MS and their family should be made aware of the importance of maintaining regular skin inspection of the person with MS. Observe the pressure points such as the sacrum and heels for redness or blanching of the skin. If this occurs advise the person to take measures to relieve the pressure.

14 Parkinson's disease

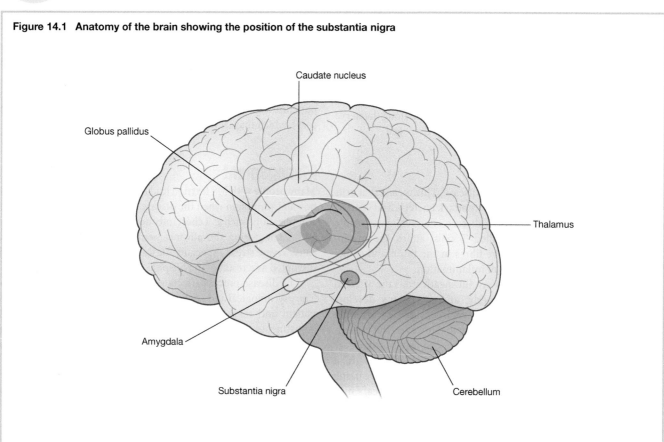

Figure 14.1 Anatomy of the brain showing the position of the substantia nigra

Caudate nucleus

Globus pallidus

Thalamus

Amygdala

Substantia nigra

Cerebellum

Overview of anatomy and physiolology

Parkinson's disease is a chronic (persistent or long-term) disorder of part of the brain. It is named after the doctor who first described it. It mainly affects the way the brain coordinates the movements of the muscles in various parts of the body. A small part of the brain called the substantia nigra (Figure 14.1) is mainly affected. This area of the brain sends messages down nerves in the spinal cord to help control the muscles of the body. Messages are passed between brain cells, nerves and muscles by chemicals called neurotransmitters. Dopamine is the main neurotransmitter that is made by the brain cells in the substantia nigra.

In Parkinson's disease, a number of cells in the substantia nigra become damaged and die. The exact cause of this is not known. Over time, more and more cells become damaged and die. As cells are damaged, the amount of dopamine that is produced is reduced. A combination of the reduction of cells and a low level of dopamine in the cells in this part of the brain causes nerve messages to the muscles to become slowed and abnormal.

Pathophysiology

A substance called dopamine acts as a messenger between two brain areas – the substantia nigra and the corpus striatum – to produce smooth, controlled movements. Most of the movement-related symptoms of Parkinson's disease are caused by a lack of dopamine, due to the loss of dopamine-producing cells in the substantia nigra. When the amount of dopamine is too low, communication between the substantia nigra and corpus striatum becomes ineffective, and movement becomes impaired; the greater the loss of dopamine, the worse the movement-related symptoms. Other cells in the brain also degenerate to some degree and may contribute to non-movement related symptoms of Parkinson's disease.

Although it is well known that lack of dopamine causes the motor symptoms of Parkinson's disease, it is not clear why the dopamine-producing brain cells deteriorate. Genetic and pathological studies have revealed that various dysfunctional cellular processes, inflammation and stress can all contribute to cell damage. In addition, abnormal clumps called Lewy bodies, which contain the protein alpha-synuclein, are found in many brain cells of individuals with Parkinson's disease. The function of these clumps in regards to Parkinson's disease is not understood. In general, scientists suspect that dopamine loss is due to a combination of genetic and environmental factors.

Signs and symptoms

The brain cells and nerves affected in Parkinson's disease normally help to produce smooth, coordinated movements of muscles. Therefore, three common Parkinson's symptoms that gradually develop are:

- **Slowness of movement** (bradykinesia). For example, it may become more of an effort to walk or to get up out of a chair. When this first develops it may be mistaken for 'getting on in years'. The diagnosis of Parkinson's disease may not become apparent unless other symptoms occur. In time, a typical walking pattern often develops. This is a 'shuffling' walk with some difficulty in starting, stopping and turning easily.
- **Stiffness of muscles** (rigidity), and muscles may feel more tense. Also, arms do not tend to swing as much when walking.
- **Shaking** (tremor) is common, but does not always occur. It typically affects the fingers, thumbs, hands and arms, but can affect other parts of the body. It is most noticeable when resting. It may become worse when anxious or emotional. It tends to become less when the hand is being used to do something such as picking up an object.

The symptoms tend slowly to become worse. However, the speed in which symptoms become worse varies from person to person. It may take several years before they become bad enough to have much effect on daily life. At first, one side of the body may be more affected than the other.

Management

Many early symptoms of Parkinson's disease can be treated by a GP, with the help of the family and other care workers in the community. The progress of the disease may vary with individuals, but should the condition of the person worsen it may be necessary to admit the person to hospital.

The nursing staff and other healthcare workers, such as the physiotherapist, speech therapist and occupational therapist should be able to advise the patient and their family on how to deal with problems interfering with activities of daily living.

As the disease process gets worse, mobility can be a problem. This includes walking, stopping walking, shuffling, tottering, falls and impaired balance. Nurses need to ensure that the person with PD is monitored all the time to prevent unnecessary injury through their unsteady gait.

Physiotherapy helps improve gait, balance and flexibility, aerobic activity and movement initiation, increase independence and provide advice about fall prevention and other safety information. Avoid walking frames (flow of movement is interrupted) unless fitted with wheels and a brake.

Occupational therapists give advice and help on maintaining all aspects relating to activities of daily living, both at work and at home, with the aim of maintaining work and family relationships, encouraging self-care where appropriate, assessing any safety issues, making cognitive assessments and arranging any appropriate interventions.

Speech therapy ensures methods of communication are available as the disease progresses and helps with swallowing difficulties (reducing the risk of aspiration).

To control symptoms of Parkinson's disease medications such as levodopa and dopamine agonists may be used.

15 Cerebrovascular accident

Figure 15.1 Blood flow through the brain

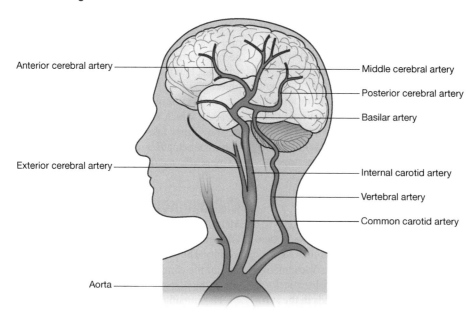

Anterior cerebral artery

Middle cerebral artery

Posterior cerebral artery

Basilar artery

Exterior cerebral artery

Internal carotid artery

Vertebral artery

Common carotid artery

Aorta

Figure 15.2 Ischaemia of brain tissue following vessel blockage

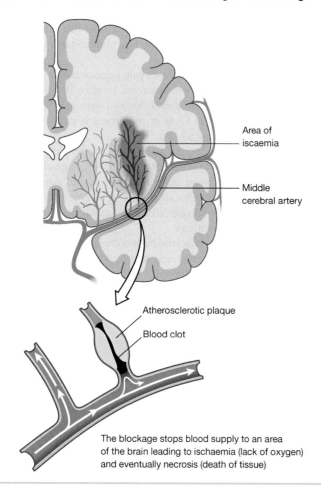

Area of iscaemia

Middle cerebral artery

Atherosclerotic plaque

Blood clot

The blockage stops blood supply to an area of the brain leading to ischaemia (lack of oxygen) and eventually necrosis (death of tissue)

Figure 15.3 Haemorrhagic stroke

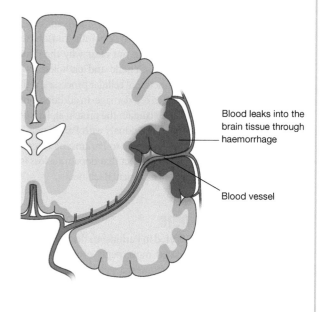

Blood leaks into the brain tissue through haemorrhage

Blood vessel

Overview of anatomy and physiology

Blood is supplied to the brain, face and scalp via two major sets of vessels: the right and left common carotid arteries and the right and left vertebral arteries (Figure 15.1).

In an adult, CBF is typically 750 millilitres per minute or 15% of the cardiac output. This equates to 50–54 millilitres of blood per 100 grams of brain tissue per minute. Too much blood (a condition known as hyperaemia) can raise ICP, which can compress and damage delicate brain tissue. Too little blood flow results if blood flow to the brain is below 18–20 ml per 100 g per minute, and tissue death occurs if flow dips below 8–10 ml per 100 g per minute.

Cerebral blood flow is determined by a number of factors, such as viscosity of blood, how dilated blood vessels are and the net pressure of the flow of blood into the brain, known as cerebral perfusion pressure, which is determined by the body's blood pressure. Cerebral blood vessels are able to change the flow of blood by altering diameters, in a process called autoregulation; they constrict when systemic blood pressure is raised and dilate when it is lowered. Arterioles also constrict and dilate in response to different chemical concentrations. For example, they dilate in response to higher levels of carbon dioxide in the blood.

Pathophysiology

A stroke is a 'brain attack' caused by sudden lack of blood supply to certain parts of the brain. This may result from a clot blocking the blood flow, narrowing of the cerebral arteries or even bursting of the blood vessels. There are two main types of stroke: ischaemic and haemorrhagic.

Ischaemic

This is the most common form of a stroke (80%), caused by blockage of blood flow to the brain by a blood clot (thrombus). Blood clots typically form in areas where the arteries have been narrowed or blocked by fatty cholesterol-containing deposits known as plaques (Figure 15.2). Another possible cause of ischaemic stroke is an irregular heartbeat (atrial fibrillation), which can cause blood clots that become lodged in the brain.

Haemorrhagic

Haemorrhagic strokes (also known as cerebral haemorrhages or intracranial haemorrhages) usually occur when a blood vessel in the brain bursts and bleeds into the brain (Figure 15.3). In about 5% of cases, the bleeding occurs on the surface of the brain (subarachnoid haemorrhage). Haemorrhagic stroke can also occur from the rupture of a balloon-like expansion of a blood vessel (aneurysm) and badly-formed blood vessels in the brain.

Signs and symptoms

A stroke (CVA) is the sudden onset of weakness, numbness, paralysis, slurred speech, aphasia, problems with vision and other manifestations of a sudden interruption of blood flow to a particular area of the brain. The ischaemic area involved determines the type of focal deficit that is seen in the patient. The FAST test is an easy way to remember the most common signs of stroke. Using the FAST test involves asking these simple questions:

Face: check their face. Has their mouth drooped?
Arm: can they lift both arms?
Speech: is their speech slurred? Do they understand you?
Time: is critical. If you see any of these signs call 999 straight away.

Other symptoms include: motor deficit depending on the area of the brain involved, causing hemiplegia or paralysis of the left or right side of the body, hemiparesis and flaccidity and spasticity; behavioural changes; communications disorders; bladder and bowel dysfunction and visual disturbances. Emotional deficits include confusion, depression and loss of control or inhibition.

Management

Management depends on the type of stroke. Treatment and care should take into account people's needs and preferences. People with acute stroke or TIA should have the opportunity, where possible, to make informed decisions about their care and treatment, in partnership with their healthcare professionals.

Good communication between healthcare professionals and people with acute stroke or TIA, as well as their families and carers, is essential. It should be supported by evidence-based written information tailored to the person's needs. Treatment and care, and the information people are given about it, should be culturally appropriate.

Medication

This may include anticoagulants, antihypertensives and statin drugs. Anticoagulants prevent blood clots by changing the chemical composition of the blood in a way that prevents clots from occurring. Heparin, warfarin and, more recently, rivaroxaban are examples of anticoagulants. Medicines that are commonly used include: thiazide diuretics, angiotensin converting enzyme (ACE) inhibitors, calcium channel blockers and beta-blockers Statins reduce the level of cholesterol in the blood by blocking an enzyme (chemical) in the liver that produces cholesterol.

Rehabilitation

After a stroke, the person may need to relearn skills and abilities, or learn new ways of doing things to adapt to the damage a stroke has caused. This is known as stroke rehabilitation. It's difficult to predict the time it will take for someone to recover from stroke, but the recovery can continue for a long time depending on the severity of the stroke.

Health professionals, for example physiotherapists, speech and language therapists, occupational therapists, ophthalmologists and psychologists, as well as doctors and nurses will work out a rehabilitation programme.

Surgery

Surgery may be performed to prevent occurrence of the stroke, to restore blood flow if the stroke has occurred and to repair vascular damage.

Prevention

This includes promoting healthy lifestyles. A low-fat, high-fibre diet is recommended, including plenty of fresh fruit and vegetables (five portions a day) and whole grains. Combining a healthy diet with regular exercise is the best way to maintain a healthy weight. Having a healthy weight reduces the chances of developing high blood pressure.

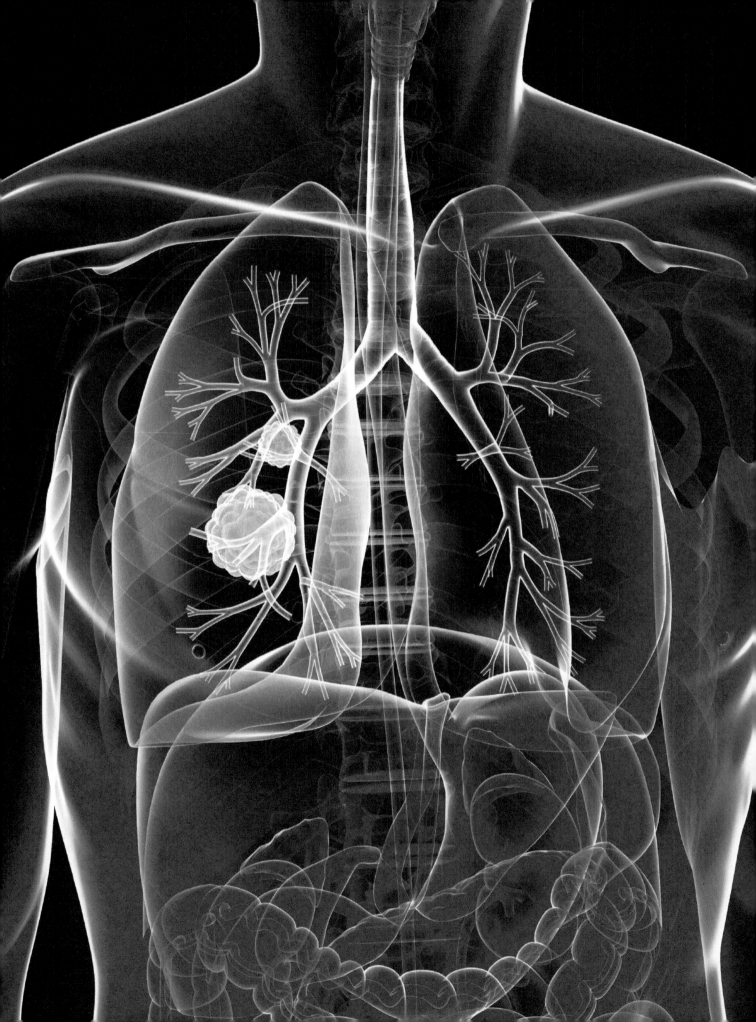

The blood

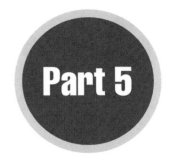

Part 5

Chapters

16 Anaemia

Figure 16.1 Components of the blood

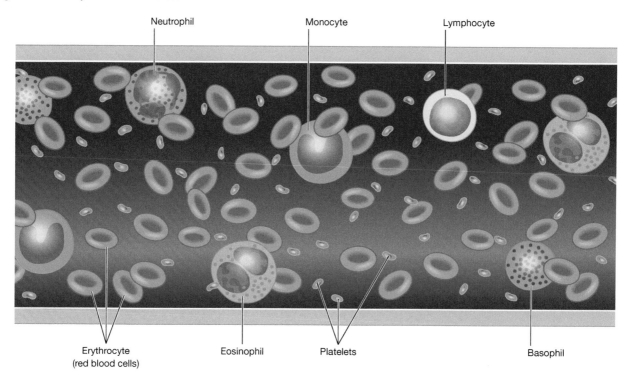

Neutrophil Monocyte Lymphocyte

Erythrocyte Eosinophil Platelets Basophil
(red blood cells)

Figure 16.2 Comparison of (a) normal and (b) iron deficiency blood smears

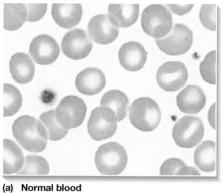 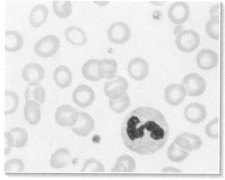

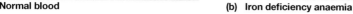

(a) Normal blood

(b) Iron deficiency anaemia

Source:
Mehta & Hoffbrand,
Haematology at a Glance, 2014

Overview of anatomy and physiology

Blood is composed of plasma and blood cells. The blood cells are erythrocytes (red blood cells), leukocytes (white blood cells) and thrombocytes (platelets). These are suspended in the plasma with other particulate matter (Figure 16.1). Plasma is a clear straw-coloured fluid that makes up more than half the volume of blood. The red blood cells and proteins contribute to the viscosity of the blood, which ranges from 3.5 to 5.5 compared with 1.000 for water. The more red blood cells and plasma proteins in blood, the higher the viscosity and the slower the flow of blood.

Plasma is the liquid part of the blood and is composed of water (91%), protein (8%) (albumin, globulin, prothrombin and fibrinogen), salts (0.9%) (sodium chloride, sodium bicarbonate and others) and the remaining 0.1% is made up of organic materials, for example fats, glucose, urea, uric acid, cholesterol and amino acids. These substances give plasma greater density and viscosity than water.

Plasma proteins make up 7% of the plasma and these proteins stay in the blood vessel as they are too large to diffuse through capillaries and are responsible for creating the osmotic pressure of blood. When plasma proteins are lost in patients who suffer from burns, fluid moves into tissues, causing oedema by a process called osmosis.

Pathophysiology

Anaemia is a condition where the amount of haemoglobin in the blood is below the normal level, or there are fewer red blood cells than normal. There are several different types of anaemia and each one has a different cause, although iron deficiency anaemia is the most common type. Other forms include vitamin B_{12} deficiency, and aplastic anaemia.

Iron deficiency anaemia

Iron deficiency anaemia occurs when there isn't enough iron in the body thus reducing the amount of red blood cells (Figure 16.2). Iron is found in meat, dried fruit and some vegetables. Iron is used by the body to make haemoglobin, which helps store and carry oxygen in red blood cells. Excess iron is stored in the liver and muscle cells, and is readily available for the production of red blood cells. Some inflammatory disorders such as Crohn's disease will affect the absorption of iron from the gastrointestinal tract, affecting the synthesis of red bloods cells.

Vitamin B_{12}/folate deficiency anaemia

Pernicious anaemia is the most common cause of vitamin B_{12} deficiency in the UK. Pernicious anaemia is an autoimmune condition affecting the stomach. An autoimmune condition means the immune system (the body's natural defence system that protects against illness and infection) attacks the body's healthy cells. Pernicious anaemia causes the immune system to attack the cells in the stomach that produce the intrinsic factor. This means the body cannot absorb vitamin B_{12}, which causes a deficiency.

Vitamin B_{12} and folate work together to help the body to produce red blood cells. Vitamin B_{12} helps to keep the nervous system (brain, nerves and spinal cord) healthy; folate is important for pregnant women because it reduces the risk of birth defects in unborn babies.

Aplastic anaemia

Aplastic anaemia is a rare, potentially life-threatening failure of haemopoiesis characterized by pancytopenia and hypocellular bone marrow. Aplastic anaemia is defined as pancytopenia with a hypocellular bone marrow in the absence of an abnormal infiltrate and with no increase in reticulin. Most cases are acquired and immune-mediated but there are also inherited forms. Environmental triggers include drugs, viruses and toxins, but most cases are idiopathic. Drugs that cause aplastic anaemia may also be related to benzene. The antibiotic, chloramphenicol and the anti-inflammatory, phenylbutazone are two examples.

What are the symptoms of aplastic anaemia?

The person complains of increasing tiredness, weakness and shortness of breath. Bleeding, bruising and blood spots may be noticed. Sore throats and other infections are noticeable. A high temperature with shivering attacks is an important symptom that demands immediate medical attention.

Signs and symptoms

Symptoms of each type of anaemia vary depending on the underlying cause of the condition. However, there are some general symptoms associated with all types of anaemia. These include: fatigue, breathlessness, lethargy, faintness, tinnitus, headache, hair loss, constipation and loss of appetite.

Management

The management of anaemia depends on which type the patient has. Iron deficiency anaemia is treated with oral iron medication and less commonly parenterally. The common medications used are ferrous gluconate and ferrous sulphate. Prior to the administration of iron medication, nurses should be aware of any drugs that may interact with iron. In syrup form the iron suspension can stain the teeth and patients should be made aware of this. Constipation, black stools and dysphagia are some of the side effects of iron tablets and therefore the patient may need laxatives to relieve the discomfort of constipation. Folic acid tablets are used to restore folate levels, which usually need to be taken for four months.

Information on food which is rich in iron should be given to patients. These include red meat, leafy vegetables and cereals. Polyphenols found in tea and coffee can impair iron absorption and therefore patients should be advised to limit these beverages until the level of iron is restored in the body. Patients who find it difficult to get enough vitamin B_{12} in their diets, such as vegans, may need vitamin B_{12} tablets for life.

17 Deep vein thrombosis

Figure 17.1   A normal vein with blood flow and a vein with a thrombus

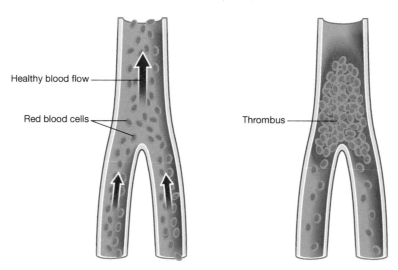

Healthy blood flow

Red blood cells

Thrombus

Figure 17.2   Capillaries

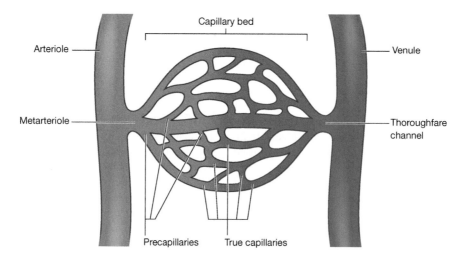

Capillary bed

Arteriole

Venule

Metarteriole

Thoroughfare channel

Precapillaries

True capillaries

Figure 17.3   Smear of blood with platelet

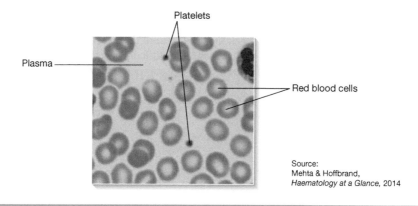

Platelets

Plasma

Red blood cells

Source:
Mehta & Hoffbrand,
Haematology at a Glance, 2014

Pathophysiology for Nurses at a Glance, First Edition. Muralitharan Nair and Ian Peate. © 2015 John Wiley & Sons, Ltd. Published 2015 by John Wiley & Sons, Ltd.
Companion website: www.ataglanceseries.com/nursing/pathophysiology

Overview of anatomy and physiology

A DVT is a blood clot in a vein. Blood clots in veins most often occur in the legs, but can occur elsewhere in the body, including the arms. The most common cause of a blood clot developing in a vein is immobility. A complication can occur in some cases where part of the blood clot breaks off and travels to the lung (pulmonary embolus).

Blood flows throughout the body tissues in blood vessels, via bulk flow (i.e. all constituents together and in one direction). The cardiovascular system is a closed-loop system, such that blood is pumped out of the heart through one set of vessels (arteries) and then returns to the heart in another (veins).

The pulmonary circulation is composed of the right heart pump and the lungs. The systemic circulation includes the left heart pump, which supplies blood to the systemic organs. The right and left heart pumps function in a series arrangement; thus both will circulate an identical volume of blood in a given minute (cardiac output: litres per minute).

In the systemic circuit, blood is ejected out of the left ventricle via a single large artery, the aorta. All arteries of the systemic circulation branch from the aorta (this is the largest artery of the body, with a diameter of 2–3 cm), and divide into progressively smaller vessels. The aorta's four principal divisions are the ascending aorta (begins at the aortic valve where, close by, the two coronary artery branches have their origin), arch of the aorta, thoracic aorta and abdominal aorta. The smallest of the arteries eventually branch into arterioles. They, in turn, branch into an extremely large number of the smallest diameter vessels, the capillaries (with an estimated 10 billion in the average human body). Next, blood exits the capillaries and begins its return to the heart via the venules.

Capillaries, which are the smallest and most numerous blood vessels in the human body (ranging from 5 to 10 micrometres in diameter and numbering around 10 billion), are also the thinnest walled vessels; an inner diameter of 5 μm is just wide enough for an erythrocyte to squeeze through (Figure 17.2).

Pathophysiology

The pathophysiology of DVT was described by Virchow in 1846 as coming from a triad of possible changes in the venous system. The triad includes changes in the vessel wall (injury), changes in the pattern of blood flow (venous stasis) and changes in the constituency of blood (hypercoagulability).

These physiological changes can occur as a result of pathology, therapies and treatments. Injury to the vessel wall may occur from trauma, surgery or invasive treatments. Patients on bedrest have venous stasis, which changes blood flow thorough the venous system, and patients on new medications may have changes in blood coagulability.

A thrombus can develop in the superficial or deep veins of the legs. The blood flow is sluggish in the affected vessels and clotting cascade takes place. Platelets aggregate at the site of injury to the vessel wall or where there is venous stasis. Platelet aggregation occurs because platelets are exposed to collagen (a protein in the connective tissue which is found in the inner surface of the blood vessel). When platelets come into contact with the exposed collagen, they release adenosine diphosphate and thromboxane. These substances make the surface of the platelets (Figure 17.3) become sticky and as they adhere to each other a platelet plug is formed. Other cells, such as the red blood cells, are trapped in the fibrin meshwork and the thrombus grows.

Signs and symptoms

Most of the time, DVT may not present with any symptoms. The possible signs and symptoms may include unexplained pyrexia and dull aching pain in the affected limb. Localized pain or tenderness within a calf or thigh muscle is a possible symptom of DVT, particularly if there is swelling in the calf below the knee or redness or warmth in that area with a heavy or aching sensation.

Management

Anticoagulant medicines prevent a blood clot from getting bigger. They can also help stop part of the blood clot from breaking off and becoming lodged in another part of the bloodstream (an embolism). Although they are often referred to as 'blood-thinning' medicines, anticoagulants do not actually thin the blood. They alter chemicals within it, which prevents clots forming so easily.

Two different types of anticoagulants are used to treat DVT: heparin and warfarin. Heparin is usually prescribed first, because it works immediately to prevent further clotting. After this initial treatment the patient may also need to take warfarin to prevent another blood clot forming.

Warfarin is taken as a tablet. It may be taken after an initial heparin treatment to prevent further blood clots occurring. It is usually recommended that warfarin is taken for 3–6 months. In some cases, warfarin may need to be taken for longer, even for life.

Compression stockings help prevent calf pain and swelling and lower the risk of ulcers developing after having a DVT. They can also help prevent post-thrombotic syndrome – damage to the tissue of the calf caused by the increase in venous pressure that occurs when a vein is blocked (by a clot) and blood is diverted to the outer veins.

18 Leukaemia

Figure 18.1 Development of blood cells from the bone marrow

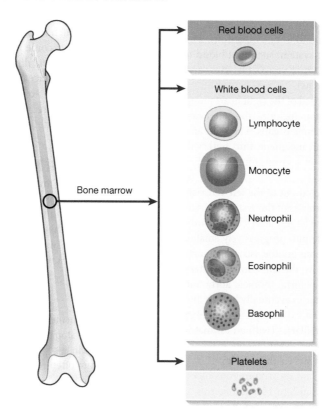

Figure 18.2 Division of stem cell into blood cells

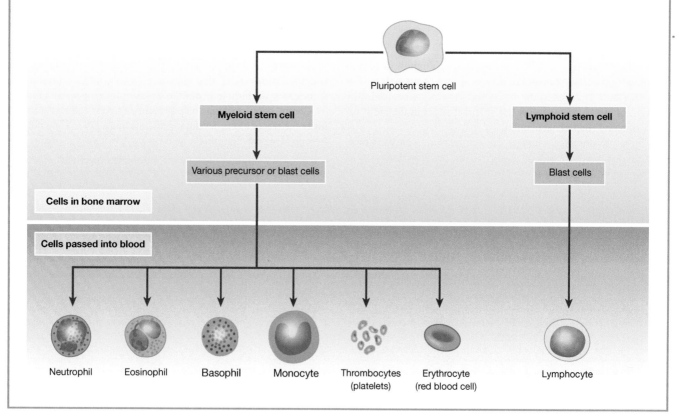

Pathophysiology for Nurses at a Glance, First Edition. Muralitharan Nair and Ian Peate. © 2015 John Wiley & Sons, Ltd. Published 2015 by John Wiley & Sons, Ltd.
Companion website: www.ataglanceseries.com/nursing/pathophysiology

Overview of anatomy and physiology

Leukaemia is a cancer of cells in the bone marrow (the cells which develop into blood cells). Leukaemia is a malignant disorder where there is an abnormal or excessive proliferation of immature white blood cells. In the UK, leukaemia is the twelfth most common cancer in adults, affecting more men than women.

All of the blood cells in the body are produced by bone marrow. Bone marrow is a spongy material found inside the bones. It is important because it produces special cells called stem cells. Stem cells are very useful because they have the ability to create other specialized cells that carry out important functions.

The large flat bones, such as the pelvis and breastbone (sternum), contain the most bone marrow. To make blood cells constantly a healthy bone marrow and nutrients from the diet are needed, including iron and certain vitamins.

Usually the bone marrow produces stem cells that are allowed to mature into 'adult' blood cells (Figure 18.1). Stem cells are primitive (immature) cells. There are two main types in the bone marrow: myeloid and lymphoid stem cells. These derive from even more primitive common 'pluripotent' stem cells (Figure 18.2). Stem cells constantly divide and produce new cells. Some new cells remain as stem cells and others go through a series of maturing stages ('precursor' or 'blast' cells) before forming into mature blood cells. Mature blood cells are released from the bone marrow into the bloodstream.

However, in cases of acute leukaemia, the affected bone marrow begins to release a large number of immature white blood cells that are known as blast cells. There are two principal types and they are acute and chronic leukaemia. Each of these is further subdivided into: acute ALL and AML and chronic CLL and CML.

Risk factors

Men are more likely to develop CML, CLL and AML than women. The risk of most leukaemias, with the exception of ALL, typically increases with age. Patients who have had certain types of chemotherapy and radiation therapy for other cancers have an increased risk of developing certain types of leukaemia.

People exposed to very high levels of radiation, such as survivors of a nuclear reactor accident, have an increased risk of developing leukaemia. Exposure to certain chemicals, such as benzene – which is found in gasoline and is used by the chemical industry – is also linked to increased risk of some kinds of leukaemia.

Pathophysiology

Acute leukaemia

Acute leukaemia is more aggressive and develops rapidly. It is more common in the younger age group; the symptoms develop quickly and if untreated become life threatening. Leukaemic cells are immature and poorly differentiated; they proliferate rapidly, have a long lifespan and do not function normally. AML is overproduction of immature myeloid white blood cells and ALL is the overproduction of immature myeloid lymphocytes called lymphoblasts. In acute leukaemia, the cells reproduce very quickly, and do not become mature enough to carry out their role in the immune system.

Acute leukaemia is characterized by a rapid increase in the number of immature blood cells. Crowding due to such cells makes the bone marrow unable to produce healthy blood cells. Acute forms of leukaemia are the most common forms of leukaemia in children.

Chronic Leukaemia

Chronic leukaemia is an uncommon type of cancer. About 600 people in the UK are diagnosed with chronic myeloid leukaemia each year. Chronic myeloid leukaemia can affect people of any age, but it is more common in people aged 40–60. There is no evidence that it runs in families.

Chronic leukaemia is characterized by the excessive build-up of relatively mature, but still abnormal, white blood cells. Typically taking months or years to progress, the cells are produced at a much higher rate than normal, resulting in many abnormal white blood cells. Whereas acute leukaemia must be treated immediately, chronic forms are sometimes monitored for some time before treatment to ensure maximum effectiveness of therapy. Chronic leukaemia mostly occurs in older people, but can theoretically occur in any age group.

Signs and symptoms

The symptoms vary depending on the exact type of leukaemia; however, the common presenting symptoms include: tiredness, breathlessness, abnormal bleeding from the gums, abdominal pain due to enlarged spleen or liver, weight loss and swollen lymph glands in the groin, neck and under the arms.

Management

Patients suffering from leukaemia will need an accurate and full assessment of pain level, activity tolerance, vital signs, nutrition, signs of bleeding or infection, in order to plan high-quality care.

Avoid situations in which trauma may occur, such as shaving with straight-edge razor, ambulating after taking medication that may cause orthostasis, or using sharp utensils. Advise the patient on the importance of maintaining hydration and taking good nutrition. Advise the patient to take frequent rests when feeling tired as fatigue is a problem for patients with leukaemia.

Adhere to local trust protocols in the care of a patient with leukaemia. Nurses must wash their hands before and after attending to the patient and discourage unnecessary visits by relatives and friends.

Pharmacological and non-pharmacological treatments

Some medications that may be prescribed include cytotoxic drugs and opioid drugs to control pain. Other interventions include radiotherapy and bone marrow transplant. Some patients may be treated with ATRA. ATRA works by changing the immature blast cells into mature healthy blood cells, and can reduce symptoms very quickly.

19 Thrombocytopenia

Figure 19.1 Blood cells

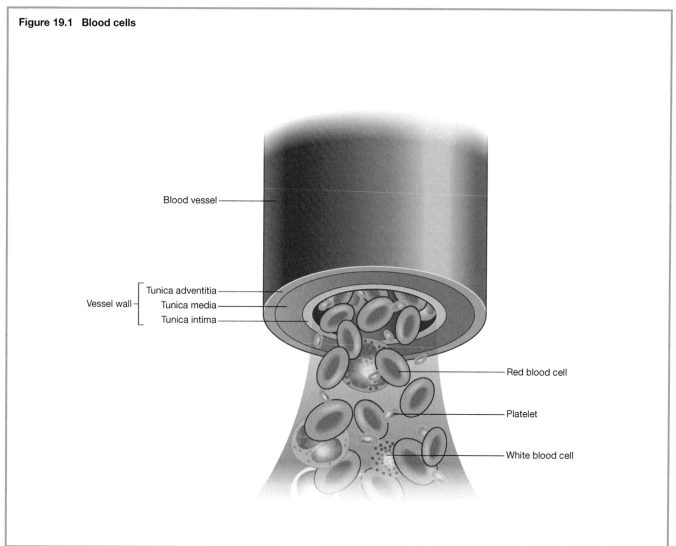

Overview of anatomy and physiology

Thrombocytopenia is the term for a reduced platelet (thrombocyte) count. It happens when platelets are lost from the circulation faster than they can be replaced from the bone marrow where they are made.

What are platelets?

Platelets are tiny cells (Figure 19.1) that circulate in the blood and whose function is to take part in the clotting process. Inside each platelet are many granules, containing compounds that enhance the ability of platelets to stick to each other and also to the surface of a damaged blood vessel wall.

The platelet count in the circulating blood is normally between 150 and 400 million per millilitre of blood. Newborn babies have a slightly lower level, but are normally within the adult range by three months of age.

Platelets are produced in the bone marrow, as are the red cells and most of the white blood cells. Platelets are produced from very large bone marrow cells called megakaryocytes. As megakaryocytes develop into giant cells, they undergo a process of fragmentation that results in the release of over 1000 platelets per megakaryocyte. The dominant hormone controlling megakaryocyte development is thrombopoietin.

Function of platelets

Platelets are essential in the formation of blood clots to prevent haemorrhage – bleeding from a ruptured blood vessel. An adequate number of normally functioning platelets is also needed to prevent leakage of red blood cells from apparently uninjured vessels.

In the event of bleeding, muscles in the vessel wall contract and reduce blood flow. The platelets then stick to each other (aggregation) and hold on to the vessel wall (primary haemostasis). The coagulation factors are then activated, resulting in normally liquid blood becoming an insoluble clot.

Pathophysiology

Three distinct types of thrombocytopenia have been identified and they are ITP, TTP and HUS. ITP is a disease in which antibodies form and destroy the body's platelets. As the destruction is believed to be caused by the body's immune system, it is therefore classified as an autoimmune disorder. Although the bone marrow increases the synthesis of platelets, it cannot keep up with the demand.

Acute ITP is more common in children, while chronic ITP is more common in adults. Acute ITP may require no treatment, especially if the platelet count does not fall too low and there is little bleeding. It usually improves spontaneously and, in children at least, rarely comes back. Chronic ITP may not need treatment if the platelet level doesn't pose a significant risk of bleeding. Any such assessment should take account of the lifestyle, such as participation in contact sports or manual work.

Platelets become coated with antibodies as a result of autoimmune response mediated by B lymphocytes. Although the platelets function normally, the spleen identifies them as foreign protein and destroys them.

TTP is a rare disease in which small blood clots form suddenly throughout the body. The numerous amounts of blood clots result in a high level of platelet usage in clotting, which leads to a reduction in platelets.

HUS is a rare disorder related to TTP in which the number of platelets decreases and there is reduction in the number of red blood cells. HUS can also occur with intestinal infections with *Escherichia coli* and with the use of some drugs, such as cyclosporine.

Drug-induced thrombocytopenia

Almost all medications can cause bad allergic reactions in sensitive people, but these reactions are rare. Drugs can also cause serious reactions with blood platelets. In these reactions, drugs stick to the platelet surface, and this combination of the drug bound to the platelet can be recognized by the body as a foreign substance and the body then makes an antibody to the drug-coated platelets, and all platelets can be destroyed.

Signs and symptoms

Thrombocytopenia symptoms may include: easy or excessive bruising, superficial bleeding into the skin that appears as a rash of petechiae, usually on the lower legs, prolonged bleeding from cuts, spontaneous bleeding from gums or nose, blood in urine or stools, unusually heavy menstrual flows and profuse bleeding during surgery or after dental work.

Management

As a result of a low level of platelets, the patient is at risk of bleeding, especially from the gums. Early identification of bleeding is important in order to prevent blood loss.

Nursing interventions include prevention, early identification and management of thrombocytopenia and its complications. Take steps to minimize the patient's risk of injury, such as preventing falls, reducing the bleeding risk and preventing infection. Be aware that thrombocytopenia increases the risk of infection in patients receiving corticosteroids. Steroid-related skin changes, bruising and bleeding under the skin increase the risk of skin breakdown. Microemboli and altered coagulation raise the risk of ischaemia of the extremities and altered organ function. To minimize these problems, ensure continuity of care and evaluate skin and organ function.

Monitor the patient's fluid intake and output to evaluate hydration status and check stools for occult blood. Remember that in thrombocytopenia, increased bleeding may lead to hypovolaemia, which can affect sensory perception and set the stage for falls and renal dysfunction. If the patient requires isolation due to immunosuppressants or infection, undertake a psychosocial assessment to evaluate psychosocial needs.

Advise the patient and family how to avoid injury. Determine the types of assistance the patient may need with activities of daily living. Advise patients and family members how to recognize signs and symptoms of infection and ischaemia.

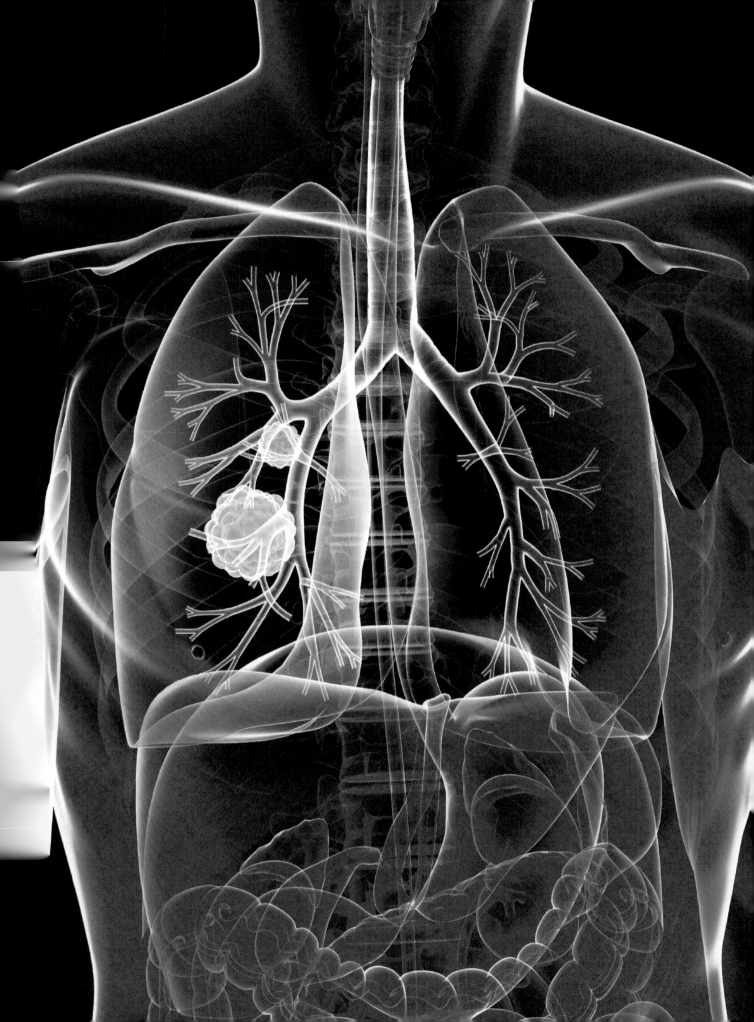

Overview of anatomy and physiology

The heart is mainly made of special muscle (myocardium). The heart pumps blood into arteries (blood vessels) which take the blood to every part of the body. Like any other muscle, the heart muscle needs a good blood supply. The coronary arteries take blood to the heart muscle (Figure 21.1). The main coronary arteries branch off from the aorta (the large artery which takes oxygen-rich blood from the heart chambers to the body.) The main coronary arteries divide into smaller branches which take blood to all parts of the heart muscle.

Pathophysiology

The most common cause of an MI is a blood clot (thrombosis) that forms inside a coronary artery, or one of its branches. This blocks the blood flow to a part of the heart. Blood clots do not usually form in normal arteries. However, a clot may form if there is some atheroma within the lining of the artery. Atheroma is like fatty patches or plaques that develop within the inside lining of arteries (Figure 21.2). (This is similar to water pipes that get furred up.) Plaques of atheroma may gradually form over a number of years in one or more places in the coronary arteries. Each plaque has an outer firm shell with a soft inner fatty core.

In an MI (heart attack), a coronary artery or one of its smaller branches is suddenly blocked, which results in the damage of the myocardium (Figure 21.3). The part of the heart muscle supplied by this artery loses its blood (and oxygen) supply if the vessel is blocked. This part of the heart muscle is at risk of dying unless the blockage is quickly removed. When a part of the heart muscle is damaged it is said to be infarcted. The term myocardial infarction (MI) means damaged heart muscle.

The area of infarct occurs in the distribution of the occluded vessel. Left main coronary artery occlusion generally results in a large anterolateral infarct, whereas occlusion of the left anterior descending coronary artery causes necrosis limited to the anterior wall. Where the infarct has taken place, a collagen scar forms in its place and the damaged muscle does not contract efficiently. Collagen is a bundle of inelastic fibres that do not stretch or contract effectively. Damaged heart tissue conducts electrical signals much more slowly than normal heart tissue, which could result in inefficient contraction of the myocardium.

Signs and symptoms

A person having an acute myocardial infarction usually has sudden chest pain that is felt behind the breast bone and sometimes travels to the left arm or the left side of the neck (Figure 21.4). Additionally, the person may have shortness of breath, sweating, nausea, vomiting, abnormal heartbeats and anxiety. Rapid, irregular pulse, hypotension and dyspnoea (shortness of breath) may all present as symptoms. The anxiety is often described as a 'sense of impending doom'. Dyspnoea occurs when the damage to the heart limits the output of the left ventricle, causing left ventricular failure and consequent pulmonary oedema.

Women experience fewer of these symptoms than men, but usually have shortness of breath, weakness, a feeling of indigestion, and fatigue. In many cases, in some estimates as high as 64%, the person does not have chest pain or other symptoms. These are called 'silent' myocardial infarctions.

Management

Patients suffering from an acute myocardial infarction will be maintained on bed rest to minimize cardiac work. Reassurance will be necessary for both the patient and relatives as they will be anxious.

Pain relief is paramount, current guidelines recommend the use of morphine (5–10 mg) or diamorphine (2.5–5 mg) titrated to pain. A popular method of titrating pain relief is to make a 10 mg dose of morphine in 10 ml of water for injection and administer the morphine in 1 ml (1 mg) increments until pain relief is achieved. The benefit of opiate pain relief is that it also acts to relieve anxiety in the patient. However, as opiates are associated with nausea and vomiting it is advisable to administer an anti-emetic at the same time. The patient is also attached to continuous cardiac monitoring as the risks of cardiac arrhythmias and even cardiac arrest are high.

Some experts still recommend the use of sublingual nitrate spray in the patient suffering from myocardial infarction. If intravenous morphine is ineffective then the recommendation is for the use of intravenous nitrates or beta blocker drugs. Before the use of nitrates or beta blockers it is necessary to measure the patient's blood pressure, as both nitrates and beta blockers can significantly reduce the blood pressure.

Pharmacological and non-pharmacological treatment

Anticoagulant, such as heparin, is commenced to minimize the risk of a thrombus developing. Drugs to dissolve clots, such as reteplase or streptokinase, are administered within two hours of developing MI to limit tissue damage. A continuous ECG monitoring is carried out to detect abnormal cardiac rhythms to take prompt action. In some patients, an emergency coronary angioplasty may be required to increase blood flow to the coronary arteries. This involves insertion of a catheter into the obstructed coronary artery under local anaesthesia. The balloon in the catheter is then inflated for 15 seconds to two or three minutes, which dilates the artery.

22 Peripheral vascular disease

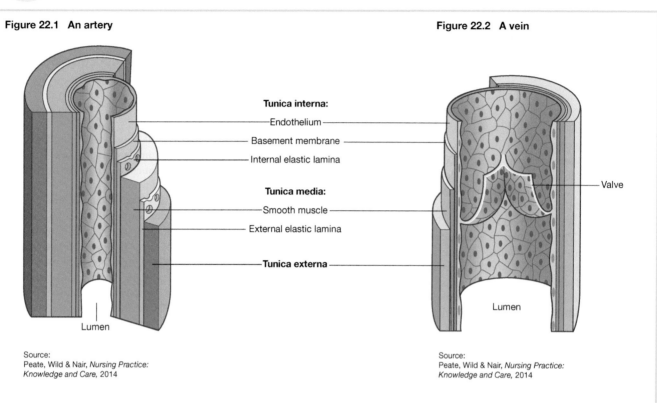

Figure 22.1   An artery

Tunica interna:
- Endothelium
- Basement membrane
- Internal elastic lamina

Tunica media:
- Smooth muscle
- External elastic lamina

Tunica externa

Lumen

Source:
Peate, Wild & Nair, *Nursing Practice: Knowledge and Care*, 2014

Figure 22.2   A vein

Valve

Lumen

Source:
Peate, Wild & Nair, *Nursing Practice: Knowledge and Care*, 2014

Figure 22.3   An artery with an atheroma

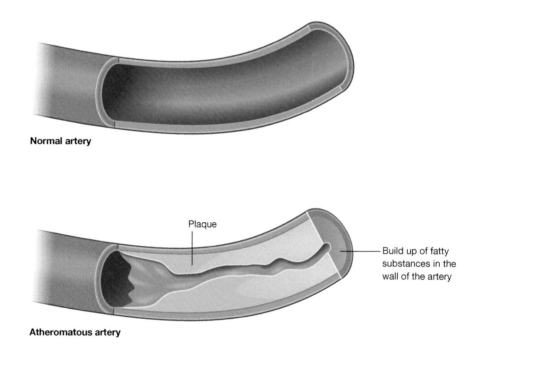

Normal artery

Plaque

Build up of fatty substances in the wall of the artery

Atheromatous artery

Overview of anatomy and physiology

Arteries and veins have the same layers of tissues in their walls, but the proportions of these layers differ. Lining the core of each is a thin layer of endothelium, and covering each is a sheath of connective tissue, but an artery has thick intermediate layers of elastic and muscular fibre, while in the vein these are much thinner and less developed. With the exception of pulmonary and umbilical veins and arteries, arteries carry oxygenated blood from the heart, while veins return deoxygenated blood to the heart.

The thicker and more muscular walls of arteries (Figure 22.1) help them to withstand and absorb the pressure waves which begin in the heart and are transmitted by the blood. The arterial wall expands and swells with the force of each contraction of the heart, then snaps back to push the blood forward as the heart rests. From the arteries, blood enters smaller branches of arteries called arterioles and then the capillary network.

Just as arterioles are smaller branches of arteries, so venules are smaller branches of veins. Venules receive blood from the capillaries and branch into veins that return blood to the heart. They do not have the need for the strength and elasticity of the arteries, so the walls of the veins are thin and almost floppy. To make up for this, many veins are located in the skeletal muscles, and the least movement of a limb squeezes the vein and drives the blood toward the heart. One-way valves ensure flow in the right direction (Figure 22.2).

Pathophysiology

PAD is a common condition in which a build-up of fatty deposits in the arteries restricts blood supply to leg muscles. It is also known as PVD. PVD is a cardiovascular disease, meaning it affects blood vessels. It is usually caused by a build-up of fatty deposits in the walls of the leg arteries. The fatty deposits, called atheroma, are made up of cholesterol and other waste substances. The narrowing of the arteries is caused by atheroma. A patch of atheroma starts quite small, and causes no problems at first. Over the years, a patch of atheroma can become thicker (Figure 22.3). (It is a bit like scale that forms on the inside of water pipes.)

What causes atheroma?

There are many risk factors associated with PVD and they include smoking, obesity, hypertension, excessive alcohol consumption, men are at higher risk than women, familial history and ethnic group (for example people who live in the UK, with ancestry from India, Pakistan, Bangladesh or Sri Lanka, have an increased risk).

Some risk factors are more risky than others. For example, smoking causes a greater risk to health than obesity. Also, risk factors interact. So, having two or more risk factors gives an increased risk compared with a person who only has one risk factor. For example, a middle-aged male smoker who does little physical activity and has a strong family history of heart disease has quite a high risk of developing a cardiovascular disease such as a heart attack, stroke or PAD before the age of 60 years.

Signs and symptoms

The typical symptom is pain, which develops in one or both calves during walking or exercise and is relieved after resting for a few minutes. This pain varies between cases and there may be aching, cramping or tiredness in the legs. This is called intermittent claudication. It is due to narrowing of one (or more) of the arteries in the leg. The most common artery affected is the femoral artery.

When walking, the calf muscles need an extra blood and oxygen supply. The narrowed artery cannot deliver the extra blood and so pain occurs from the oxygen-starved muscles. The pain comes on more rapidly when walking up a hill or stairs than when on the flat. If an artery higher upstream is narrowed, such as the iliac artery or aorta, then the person may develop pain in the thighs or buttocks when they walk.

If the blood supply is very much reduced, then the person may develop pain even at rest, particularly at night when the legs are raised in bed. Typically, rest pain first develops in the toes and feet rather than in the calves. Ulcers (sores) may develop on the skin of the feet or lower leg if the blood supply to the skin is poor. In a small number of cases, gangrene (death of tissue) of a foot may result.

Management

Pain control is paramount in patients with arterial insufficiency. If pain is caused by exercise, such as walking long distances, then they should be advised against it. However, light exercise which they can tolerate should be encouraged as it helps to improve circulation. Patients should be advised to keep themselves warm if they are affected by cold weather, but they should avoid tight fitting clothing, smoking, cold temperatures and sitting crossed-legged for too long.

Patients may need medications such as beta blockers, anticoagulants, lipid-lowering drugs and antiplatelet drugs. NICE recommends naftidrofuryl oxalate for the treatment of intermittent claudication for PAD. Naftidrofuryl oxalate improves blood flow in the body.

Surgery

There are two main types of surgical treatment for PAD: angioplasty – where a blocked or narrowed section of artery is widened by inflating a tiny balloon inside the vessel; and bypass graft – where blood vessels are taken from another part of the body and used to bypass the blockage in an artery

Angina

Figure 23.1   Blockage of the coronary artery

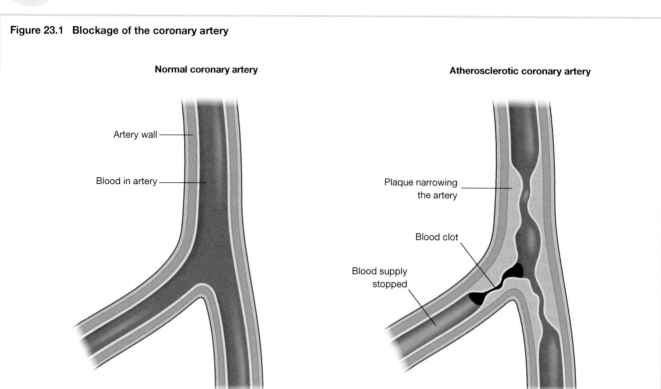

Normal coronary artery

- Artery wall
- Blood in artery

Atherosclerotic coronary artery

- Plaque narrowing the artery
- Blood clot
- Blood supply stopped

Overview of anatomy and physiology

Angina is a pain that comes from the heart. It is usually caused by narrowing of the coronary (heart) arteries (Figure 23.1). Usual treatment includes a statin medicine to lower cholesterol level, low-dose aspirin to help prevent a heart attack and a beta blocker medicine to help protect the heart and to prevent angina pains.

The heart is mainly made of special muscle. The heart pumps blood into arteries which take the blood to every part of the body. Like any other muscle, the heart muscle needs a good blood supply. The coronary arteries take blood to the heart muscle. They are the first arteries to branch off the aorta. This is the large artery taking blood from the heart to the rest of the body. In angina, one or more of the coronary arteries is usually narrowed. This causes a reduced blood supply to a part, or parts, of the heart muscle.

Pathophysiology

Angina pain closely resembles the signs and symptoms of MI; thus it is vital that carers are able to differentiate between the two conditions, as the treatment differs in both cases. If a patient has angina pain, this is usually relived by vasodilators, for example GTN, but the angina pain is rarely fatal.

Angina results from a blockage in the coronary arteries, giving diminished blood supply to the affected part of the heart muscle. At rest the blood supply may be sufficient to provide nutrients and oxygen to the heart muscle; however, during activity, for example walking or running, the heart rate increases, which puts more effort on the heart. During exertion, if the blood flow to the heart muscle is inadequate, the oxygen supply is also diminished, leading to severe pain. The patient may present with pallor, dyspnoea, cyanosis, diaphoresis and tachycardia.

Types of angina

Stable angina

This is the most common type of angina, and pain is usually brought about by physical exertion that results in the heart rate increasing. This type of angina is defined as stable because there is a regular pattern for the pain and similar triggers exist for each attack of angina. Sufferers of stable angina can usually predict how an attack can happen, and these attacks usually only last for a couple of minutes. The pain is usually relieved by rest or by taking angina medication

Unstable angina

Unstable angina does not follow a regular pattern. A small amount of physical effort such as walking, or even just resting, can result in an attack. In many cases, stable angina can progress to unstable angina, which may be an indication of worsening of coronary heart disease. In these cases, you should see a doctor urgently. Generally, pain from unstable angina is worse than with stable angina. The pain also tends to happen more often, and each episode may last as long as half an hour.

Variant angina

Variant angina is a rare form of angina. It is thought to occur as a result of coronary artery vasospasm, resulting in diminished blood flow. Variant angina is very painful and occurs from midnight to early morning. It usually occurs at rest and the same time each day.

Signs and symptoms

The primary symptom of angina is chest pain, which is usually described as a 'heaviness' or a feeling of 'pressure' on the chest cavity. Severity of this pain varies from person to person, and patients can experience anything from a dull ache to severe pain. Sometimes angina pain may extend from the chest to the neck, down the arm and into the stomach, back, or jaw. In addition to the pain in these areas, other angina symptoms can include breathlessness, sweating and nausea.

Angina symptoms develop when the heart demands more blood than is supplied to it by the coronary arteries. This increased demand for blood is usually brought on by physical activity, but can also include other triggers such as emotional upset, stress, cold weather or after a meal. Depending on the type of angina, symptoms usually last less than ten minutes once the person has stopped the activity that triggered the pain.

Management

Healthcare professionals play a crucial role in the management of patients with angina. An accurate assessment of the patient must be carried out to ascertain the location, duration and the intensity of the pain. Risk factors must be identified to provide high-quality care. The care should include controlling pain, reducing anxiety and providing information on the possible risk factors and how to take appropriate measures to minimize the risk of developing angina.

The main goals of treatment in angina pectoris are to relieve the symptoms, slow the progression of disease and reduce the possibility of future events, especially MI and premature death.

Smoking cessation results in a significant reduction of acute adverse effects on the heart and may reverse, or at least slow, atherosclerosis. Strongly encourage patients to quit smoking, and take an active role in helping them to achieve this goal.

Pharmacological interventions

A beta blocker or a calcium channel blocker is used as first-line treatment for stable angina. The choice of the drug to use is based on comorbidities, contraindications and the person's preference.

Coronary revascularization

Coronary revascularization is required in those at high risk and those who fail to be controlled by medical therapy. A cardiac rehabilitation programme should be arranged following revascularization. Both coronary artery bypass grafting and percutaneous transluminal angioplasty have their indications and advocates. For the low-risk patient with stable angina, medical management carries the lowest risk.

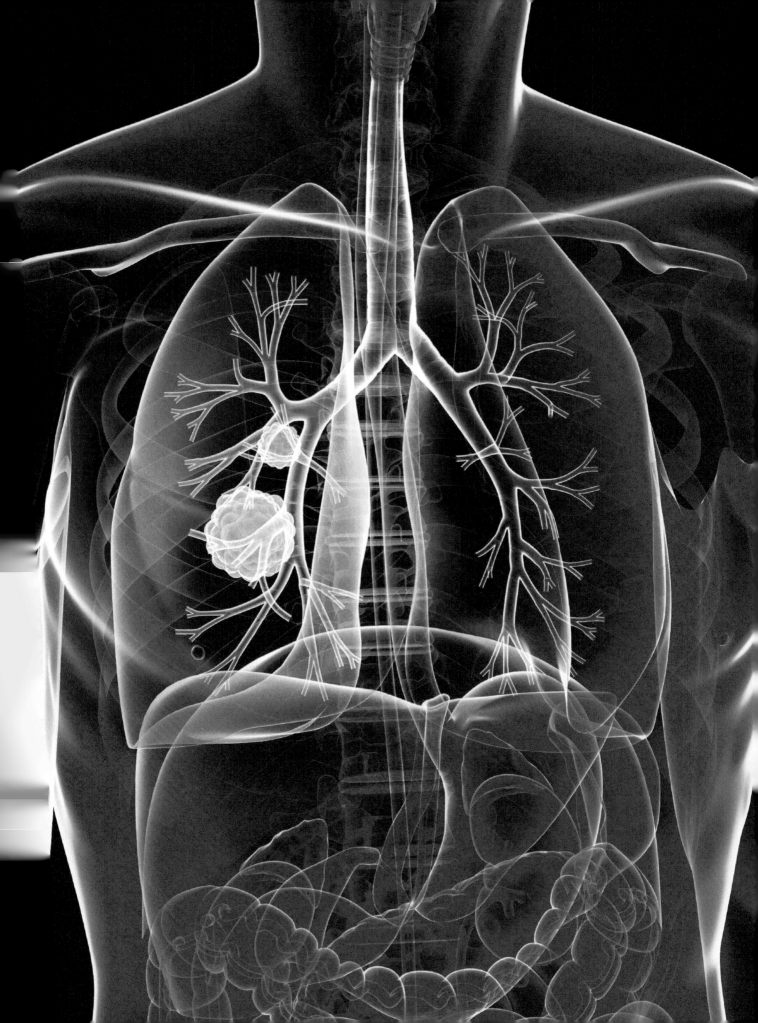

The respiratory system

Part 7

Chapters

24 Asthma

Figure 24.1   Bronchial tree

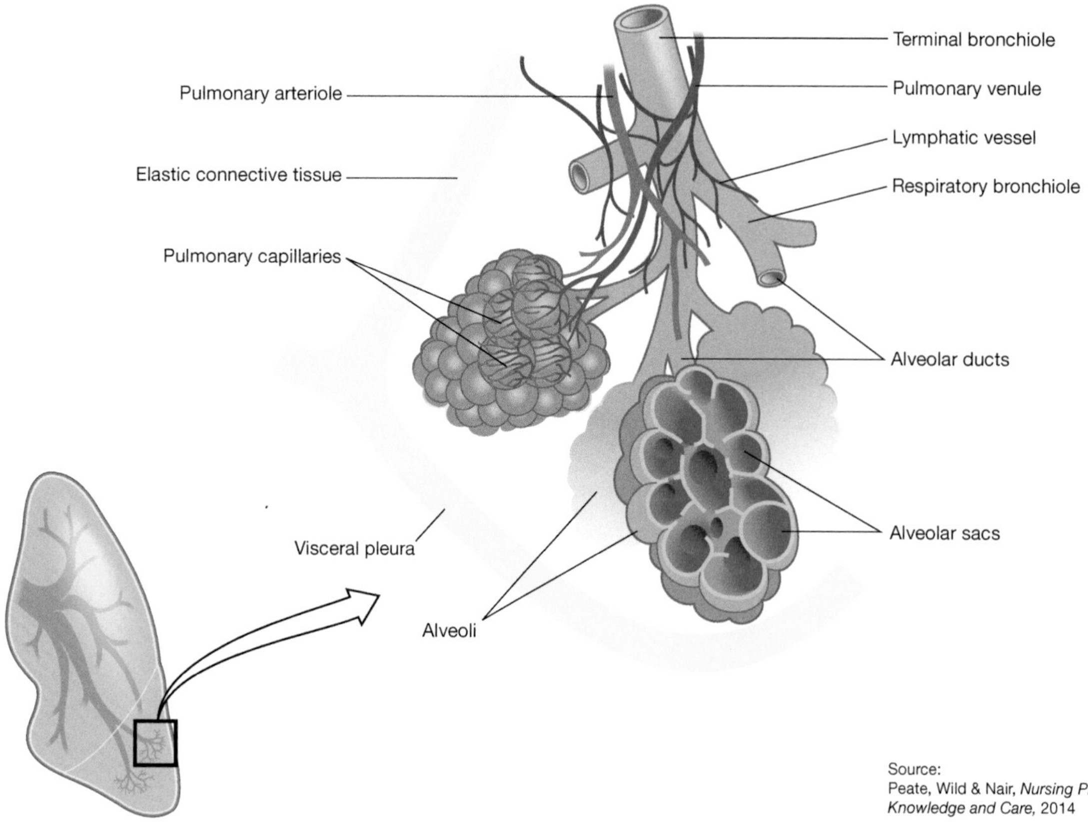

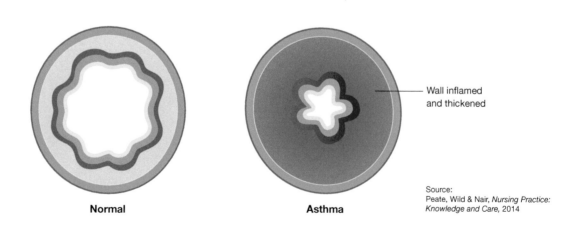

Terminal bronchiole

Pulmonary arteriole

Pulmonary venule

Lymphatic vessel

Elastic connective tissue

Respiratory bronchiole

Pulmonary capillaries

Alveolar ducts

Alveolar sacs

Visceral pleura

Alveoli

Source:
Peate, Wild & Nair, *Nursing Practice:
Knowledge and Care,* 2014

Figure 24.2   Changes in the bronchioles in asthma

Wall inflamed
and thickened

Source:
Peate, Wild & Nair, *Nursing Practice:
Knowledge and Care,* 2014

Normal

Asthma

Pathophysiology for Nurses at a Glance, First Edition. Muralitharan Nair and Ian Peate. © 2015 John Wiley & Sons, Ltd. Published 2015 by John Wiley & Sons, Ltd.
Companion website: www.ataglanceseries.com/nursing/pathophysiology

Overview of anatomy and physiology

Asthma is caused by inflammation of the airways. These are the small tubes, called bronchi, which carry air in and out of the lungs. In asthma, the bronchi will be inflamed and more sensitive than normal.

The airways of the lungs consist of the cartilaginous bronchi, membranous bronchi and gas-exchanging bronchi, termed the respiratory bronchioles and alveolar ducts (Figure 24.1). While the first two types function mostly as anatomic dead space, they also contribute to airway resistance. The smallest non-gas-exchanging airways, the terminal bronchioles, are approximately 0.5 mm in diameter; airways are considered small if they are less than 2 mm in diameter.

Cellular elements include mast cells, which are involved in the complex control of releasing histamine and other mediators. Basophils, eosinophils, neutrophils and macrophages also are responsible for extensive mediator release in the early and late stages of bronchial asthma. Stretch and irritant receptors reside in the airways, as do cholinergic motor nerves, which innervate the smooth muscle and glandular units. In bronchial asthma, smooth muscle contraction in an airway is greater than that expected for its size if it were functioning normally, and this contraction varies in its distribution.

Pathophysiology

Some of the principal cells identified in airway inflammation include mast cells, eosinophils, epithelial cells, macrophages and activated T lymphocytes. T lymphocytes play an important role in the regulation of airway inflammation through the release of numerous cytokines. Other constituent airway cells, such as fibroblasts, endothelial cells and epithelial cells, contribute to the chronicity of the disease. Other factors, such as adhesion molecules (e.g. selectins, integrins), are critical in directing the inflammatory changes in the airway. Finally, cell-derived mediators influence smooth muscle tone and produce structural changes and remodelling of the airway.

The presence of airway hyper-responsiveness or bronchial hyper-reactivity in asthma is an exaggerated response to numerous exogenous and endogenous stimuli. The mechanisms involved include direct stimulation of airway smooth muscle and indirect stimulation by pharmacologically active substances from mediator-secreting cells such as mast cells or non-myelinated sensory neurons. The degree of airway hyper-responsiveness generally correlates with the clinical severity of asthma.

Airway obstruction causes increased resistance to airflow and decreased expiratory flow rates. These changes lead to a decreased ability to expel air and may result in hyperinflation (Figure 24.2). The resulting over-distention helps maintain airway patency, thereby improving expiratory flow; however, it also alters pulmonary mechanics and increases the work of breathing.

Bronchial hyper-responsiveness

Hyperinflation compensates for the airflow obstruction, but this compensation is limited when the tidal volume approaches the volume of the pulmonary dead space; the result is alveolar hypoventilation. Uneven changes in airflow resistance, the resulting uneven distribution of air, and alterations in circulation from increased intra-alveolar pressure due to hyperinflation all lead to ventilation-perfusion mismatch. Vasoconstriction due to alveolar hypoxia also contributes to this mismatch. Vasoconstriction is also considered an adaptive response to ventilation/perfusion mismatch.

Signs and symptoms

The symptoms of asthma can range from mild to severe. When asthma symptoms get significantly worse, it is known as an asthma attack. The symptoms include feeling breathless, a tight chest, like a band tightening around it, wheezing, which makes a whistling sound when the patient breathes, coughing, particularly at night, and early morning attacks triggered by exercise, exposure to allergens and other triggers.

A severe asthma attack usually develops slowly, taking 6–48 hours to become serious. However, for some people, asthma symptoms can get worse quickly.

What causes asthma symptoms to occur?

Many things can trigger or worsen asthma symptoms. A doctor will help a patient find out which things (called triggers) may cause asthma to flare up if there is contact with them. Triggers can include: allergens from dust, animal fur, cockroaches, mould, and pollens from trees, grasses and flowers, irritants such as cigarette smoke, air pollution, chemicals or dust in the workplace, compounds in home decor products, sprays (such as hairspray), medicines (such as aspirin or other non-steroidal anti-inflammatory drugs and non-selective beta blockers), viral upper respiratory infections (such as colds) and chemicals in food and drinks.

Management

The aim of treatment is to get asthma under control and keep it that way. Everyone with asthma should be able to lead a full and unrestricted life. The treatments available for asthma are effective in most people and should enable them to be free from symptoms. These should include: continuous monitoring of vital signs until the patient is stabilized, and safe administration of prescribed oxygen and medications.

Regular PEFR measurement – singular or infrequent peak flows will not accurately reflect the patient's status. PEFR should be measured every 15–30 minutes after commencement of treatment until conditions stabilize. PEFR can also be used to measure the effectiveness of bronchodilator therapy; therefore, PEFR should be measured pre- and post-inhaled or nebulized beta-2 agonists at least four times a day throughout their stay in hospital.

Health promotion – avoidance of triggers, compliance with prescribed pharmacological therapies, smoking cessation and weight reduction in obese patients may reduce the frequency of asthma attacks.

25 Chronic bronchitis

Figure 25.1 Respiratory system

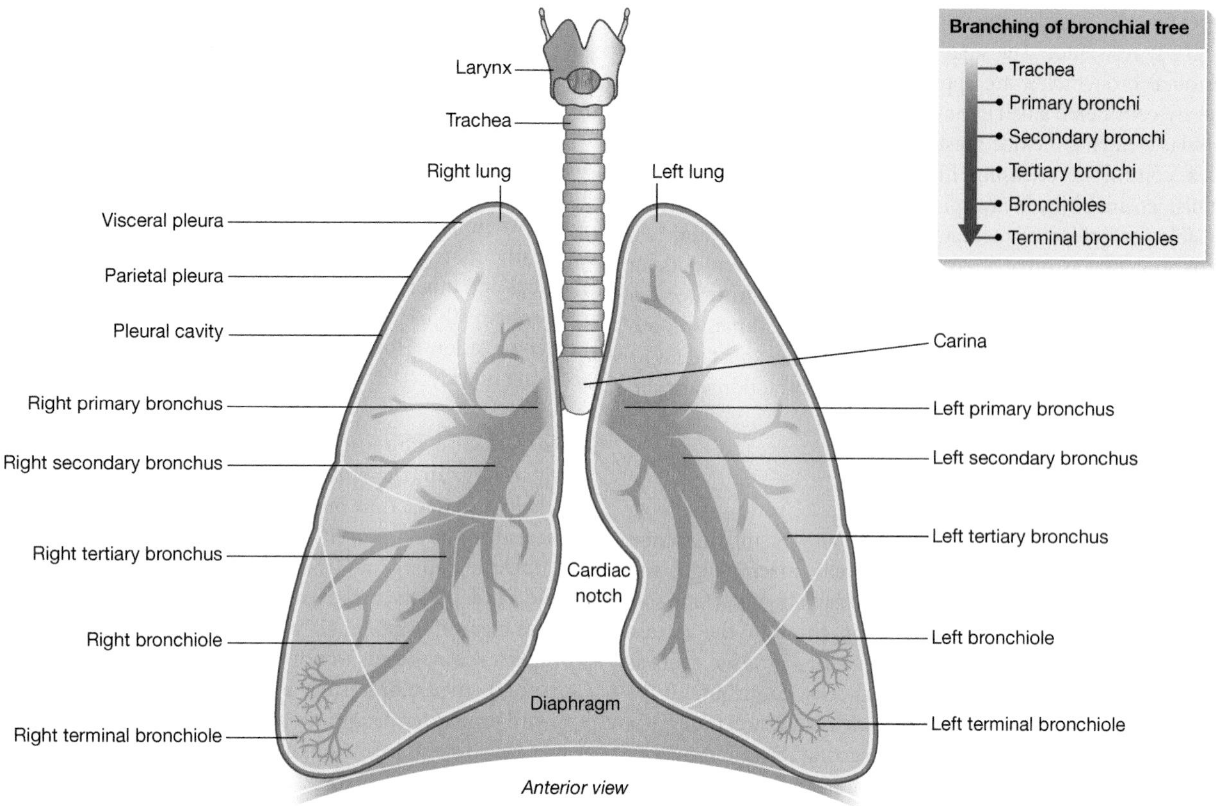

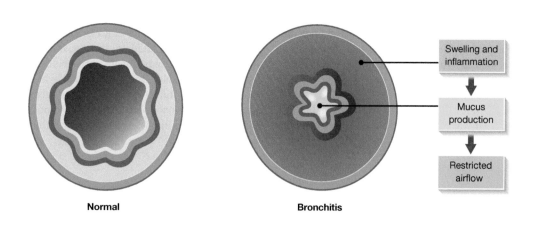

Larynx

Trachea

Right lung

Left lung

Visceral pleura

Parietal pleura

Pleural cavity

Carina

Right primary bronchus

Left primary bronchus

Right secondary bronchus

Left secondary bronchus

Right tertiary bronchus

Left tertiary bronchus

Cardiac notch

Right bronchiole

Left bronchiole

Diaphragm

Right terminal bronchiole

Left terminal bronchiole

Anterior view

Branching of bronchial tree

- Trachea
- Primary bronchi
- Secondary bronchi
- Tertiary bronchi
- Bronchioles
- Terminal bronchioles

Source:
Peate, Wild & Nair, *Nursing Practice: Knowledge and Care*, 2014

Figure 25.2 Narrowing of the inflamed bronchial tube

Normal

Bronchitis

Swelling and inflammation

↓

Mucus production

↓

Restricted airflow

Pathophysiology for Nurses at a Glance, First Edition. Muralitharan Nair and Ian Peate. © 2015 John Wiley & Sons, Ltd. Published 2015 by John Wiley & Sons, Ltd.
Companion website: www.ataglanceseries.com/nursing/pathophysiology

Overview of anatomy and physiology

The upper respiratory tract consists of the oral cavity (mouth), the nasal cavity (the nose), the pharynx and the larynx. As well as providing smell and speech the upper respiratory tract ensures that the air entering the lower respiratory tract is warm, damp and clean.

The lower respiratory tract includes the trachea, the right and left primary bronchi and the constituents of both lungs (Figure 25.1). The trachea (or windpipe) is a tubular vessel that carries air from the larynx down towards the lungs. The trachea is also lined with pseudostratified ciliated columnar epithelium so that any inhaled debris are trapped and propelled upwards towards the oesophagus and pharynx to be swallowed or expectorated. The trachea and the bronchi also contain irritant receptors, which stimulate coughs, forcing larger invading particles upwards.

The bronchi are the main airways in the lungs, which branch off on either side of the windpipe (trachea). They lead to smaller and smaller airways inside the lungs, known as bronchioles (Figure 25.1). The walls of the bronchi produce mucus to trap dust and other particles that could otherwise cause irritation.

The nasal cavity is also lined with a mucus membrane made from pseudostratified ciliated columnar epithelium, which contains a network of capillaries and a plentiful supply of mucus-secreting goblet cells.

Pathophysiology

Cells that line the airways in the lungs normally produce mucus as part of the body's defence mechanism against bacteria, viruses and other foreign particles. The mucus traps these particles, and tiny hair-like projections in the airways (called cilia) sweep the dirty mucus up and out of the lungs.

Many of the bronchi develop chronic inflammation with swelling and excess mucus production (Figure 25.2). The inflammation causes a change in the lining cells of the airways to varying degrees. Many cells that line the airway lose the function of their cilia (hair-like appendages that are capable of beating rapidly), and eventually the ciliated cells are lost. Cilia perform the function of moving particles and fluid (usually mucus) over the lining surface in such structures as the trachea, bronchial tubes and nasal cavities, to keep these hollow structures clear of particles and fluids. These ciliated cells that help in clearance of secretions are often replaced by so-called goblet cells. This group of cells secretes mucus into the airway. The warm moist environment of the airway, along with the nutrients in the mucus, are an excellent medium for growing bacteria. The mucus often becomes infected and discoloured from the bacterial overgrowth and the body's inflammatory response to it. The inflammation, swelling and mucus frequently and significantly inhibit the airflow to and from the lung alveoli by narrowing and partially obstructing the bronchi and bronchioles.

The muscles that surround some of the airways can be stimulated by this airway irritation. This muscular spasm, also known as bronchospasm, can result in further airway narrowing.

In chronic bronchitis, more mucus than normal is constantly produced. This causes a build-up of excess mucus that the cilia are unable to clear from the lungs. Exacerbating this is the fact that the cilia become dysfunctional and are less efficient at expelling mucus from the lungs. The build-up of mucus narrows the airways and provides havens for bacteria to thrive, leading to more frequent and serious lung infections, and even more mucus production.

In chronic bronchitis there is a long-lasting cough and mucus production. The airways in the lungs become swollen and produce more mucus.

Signs and symptoms

Cough and sputum production are the most common symptoms; they usually last for at least three months and occur daily. The intensity of coughing and the amount and frequency of sputum production varies from patient to patient. Sputum may be clear, yellowish, greenish or, occasionally, blood-tinged. Since cigarette smoke is the most common cause of chronic bronchitis, it should not be surprising that the most common presentation is so-called smoker's cough. This is characterized by a cough that tends to be worse on getting up and is often productive of discoloured mucus in the early part of the day. As the day progresses, less mucus is produced. The person may also present with wheezing, and dyspnoea often occurs.

Management

The key point with regards to the management is to avoid the triggers that cause chronic bronchitis. For patients with an acute exacerbation of chronic bronchitis, therapy with short-acting agonists or anticholinergic bronchodilators should be administered during the acute exacerbation. In addition, a short course of systemic corticosteroid therapy may be given and has been proven to be effective.

Smoking causes bronchoconstriction and paralyses the cilia, the tiny, protective hairs that line the airways. Because cilia are important in removing irritating substances and particles from the lungs, damage to them results in difficulty or an inability to remove secretions. Smokers are also more susceptible to lung infections, which are a common problem for people with chronic bronchitis.

Unless contraindicated, patients should be advised to have flu vaccines yearly. Patients with CB are prone to chest infection and thus when they have flu they are at risk of developing a chest infection.

Advise on simple measures such as getting plenty of rest, drinking lots of fluids, avoiding smoke and fumes, and possibly getting a prescription for an inhaled bronchodilator and/or cough medicines.

Pulmonary embolism

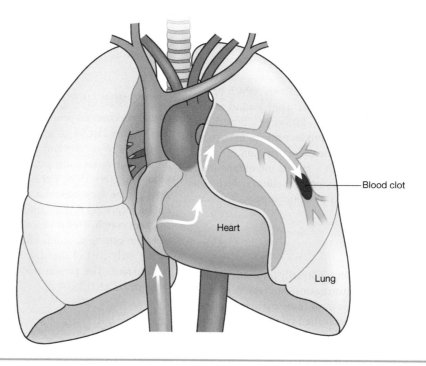

Figure 26.1 Formation of a pulmonary embolism: a blood clot from the leg vein, travels to the heart and then becomes lodged in a blood vessel (artery) in the lungs

Blood clot

Heart

Lung

Pathophysiology for Nurses at a Glance, First Edition. Muralitharan Nair and Ian Peate. © 2015 John Wiley & Sons, Ltd. Published 2015 by John Wiley & Sons, Ltd.
Companion website: www.ataglanceseries.com/nursing/pathophysiology

Overview of anatomy and physiology

A pulmonary embolism (PE) is a blockage in the pulmonary artery, which is the blood vessel that carries blood from the heart to the lungs. This blockage, usually a blood clot, is potentially life threatening as it can prevent the blood from reaching the lungs. A small proportion of cases are due to the embolization of air, fat or talc in drugs of intravenous drug abusers and a small piece of tumour (cancer) that has broken off from a larger tumour in the body.

Small clots may cause no symptoms at all and medium ones cause sudden breathlessness. Sometimes, if a clot is big enough to block lung circulation, it can cause collapse or even sudden death. Smaller wandering clots can break off a clot in the leg over several days. This causes increasingly troublesome symptoms. The lungs can start to bleed temporarily, which causes sharp pains when the patient breathes. The patient can also cough up blood.

Pathophysiology

A PE is a blockage in one of the arteries (blood vessels) in the lungs, usually due to a blood clot. A PE can be in an artery in the centre of the lung or one near the edge of the lung. The clot can be large or small and there can be more than one clot. If there are severe symptoms, which occur with a large clot near the centre of the lung, this is known as a massive PE, and is very serious.

A massive PE is so called not due to the actual size of the embolus (blood clot) but due to the size of its effect. A PE is high risk if it causes serious problems such as a collapse or low blood pressure. Massive PEs are, by definition, high risk. About one in seven people with a massive PE will die as a result.

In almost all cases, the cause is a blood clot (thrombus) that has originally formed in a deep vein (known as a DVT). This clot travels through the circulation and eventually gets stuck in one of the blood vessels in the lung. The thrombus that has broken away is called an embolus (and can therefore cause an embolism). Most DVTs come from veins in the legs or pelvis. Occasionally, a PE may come from a blood clot in an arm vein, or from a blood clot formed in the heart.

Blood vessel damage

If a blood vessel is damaged, the inside of the blood vessel can become narrowed or blocked. This can result in a blood clot forming.

Blood vessels can be damaged by injuries such as broken bones or severe muscle damage. If a blood vessel is damaged during surgery, a blood clot may develop, particularly in operations that are carried out on the lower half of the body. Conditions such as vasculitis and some types of medication, such as chemotherapy medication, can also lead to blood vessel damage.

How is it diagnosed?

Because the severity of the disease is extremely varied and all the symptoms are common in other conditions, diagnosis can be difficult. Various tests may be used to help confirm the diagnosis. These may include one or more of the following: ultrasound of the leg, blood test for D-dimer and isotope scan, and CTPA scan.

Signs and symptoms

Symptoms of PE are typically sudden in onset and include dyspnoea (difficulty in breathing), tachypnoea (rapid breathing), chest pain of a 'pleuritic' nature (worsened by breathing), cough and haemoptysis (coughing up blood). A PE can cause symptoms such as chest pain or breathlessness, but may have no symptoms and be hard to detect.

More severe cases can include signs such as cyanosis, collapse and circulatory instability, due to decreased blood flow through the lungs and into the left side of the heart.

A massive pulmonary embolism can cause collapse and death.

Management

Anticoagulation is often called thinning of the blood. However, it does not actually thin the blood. It alters certain chemicals in the blood to stop clots forming so easily. It doesn't dissolve the clot either (as some people incorrectly think). Anticoagulation prevents a PE from getting larger, and prevents any new clots from forming. The body's own healing mechanisms can then get to work to break up the clot. Anticoagulation treatment is usually started immediately (as soon as a PE is suspected) in order to prevent the clot worsening, while waiting for test results.

The main anticoagulants used to treat pulmonary embolisms are low molecular weight heparin (LMWH) and warfarin. Low molecular weight heparin is given as an injection. Regular injections of this medication are usually used as the initial treatment for a pulmonary embolism because they start working immediately.

Warfarin comes in tablet form, which is usually taken soon after the initial treatment with LMWH. Warfarin takes longer to start working than heparin injections, but as it is more convenient to take it is usually recommended for a longer period after the patient has stopped having these injections.

Treatment with warfarin will usually be recommended for at least three months, although some patients need to take it for longer than this. Occasionally, patients may need to take warfarin for the rest of their life.

Other considerations include bed rest during treatment, compression stockings, advice on the cessation of smoking, diet and exercise, and maintaining a healthy weight.

27 Chronic obstructive pulmonary disease

Figure 27.1   Normal lung and a lung with bronchial stricture (arrowed)

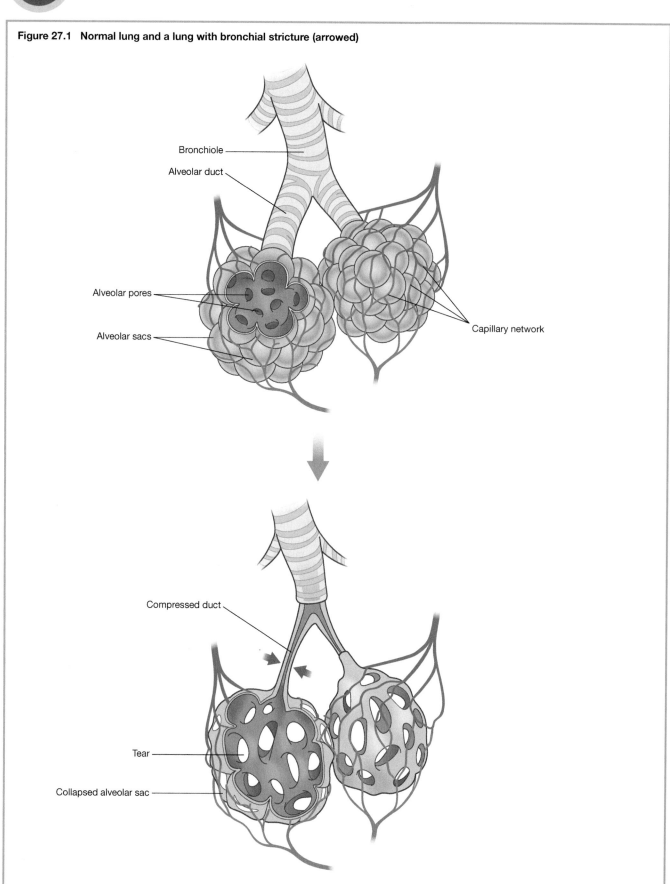

Bronchiole

Alveolar duct

Alveolar pores

Alveolar sacs

Capillary network

Compressed duct

Tear

Collapsed alveolar sac

Overview of anatomy and physiology

Chronic obstructive pulmonary disease (COPD) is the name for a collection of lung diseases including chronic bronchitis, emphysema and chronic obstructive airways disease. COPD affects middle-aged and older adults. For the anatomy and physiology of the respiratory system see Part 5 of *Anatomy and Physiology at a Glance*.

Pathophysiology

COPD is characterized by slow progressive obstruction of the airways. COPD is a condition where the airways become inflamed and the air sacs in the lungs are damaged. This causes the airways to become narrower (Figure 27.1), which makes it harder to breathe in and out.

The most consistent pathophysiological finding is hypertrophy and an increase in number of the mucus secreting goblet cells of the bronchial tree, evenly distributed throughout the lung but mainly seen in the larger bronchi.

The small airways are particularly affected early in the disease, initially without the development of any significant breathlessness. This initial inflammation of the small airways is reversible and accounts for the improvement in airway function if smoking is stopped early. In later stages the inflammation continues even if smoking is stopped. Further progression of the disease leads to progressive squamous cell metaplasia and fibrosis of the bronchial walls.

The physiological consequence of these changes is the development of airflow limitation. If the airway narrowing is combined with emphysema (causing loss of the elastic recoil of the lung with collapse of small airways during aspiration) the resulting airflow limitation is even more severe. As the air sacs get permanently damaged, it will become increasingly difficult to breathe out.

Causes of COPD

Smoking is the main cause of COPD. At least four out of five people who develop the disease are, or have been, smokers. The lining of the airways becomes inflamed and permanently damaged by smoking. This damage cannot be reversed. Around 10–25% of smokers develop COPD.

Exposure to certain types of dust and chemicals at work, including grains, isocyanates, cadmium and coal, has been linked to the development of COPD, even in people who do not smoke. Air pollution may be an additional risk factor for COPD.

There is a rare genetic tendency to develop COPD, called alpha-1-antitrypsin deficiency. This causes COPD in a small number of people (about 1%). Alpha-1-antitrypsin is a protein that protects the lungs. Without it, the lungs can be damaged by other enzymes that occur naturally in the body. People who have an alpha-1-antitrypsin deficiency usually develop COPD at a younger age, often under 35.

Signs and symptoms

The symptoms of COPD usually develop over a number of years, so the person may not be aware that they have the condition. The patient may have:

- Increasing breathlessness when exercising or moving around
- A persistent cough with phlegm that never seems to go away
- Frequent chest infections, particularly in winter
- Wheezing

Symptoms of COPD are often worse in winter, and it is common to have two or more flare-ups a year. A flare-up (also known as an exacerbation) is when the symptoms are particularly bad. This is one of the most common reasons for people being admitted to hospital in the UK.

Chest infections are more common if the person has COPD. Wheezing with cough and breathlessness may become worse than usual if the person has a chest infection and the person may cough more sputum. Sputum usually turns yellow or green during a chest infection. Chest infections can be caused by bacteria **or** viruses. Bacteria (which can be killed using antibiotics) cause about one in two or three exacerbations of COPD. Viruses (which cannot be killed with antibiotics) are a common cause of exacerbations too, particularly in the winter months. The common cold virus may be responsible for up to one in three exacerbations.

Other signs of COPD can include:

- Weight loss
- Tiredness and fatigue
- Swollen ankles

Management

There is no cure for COPD, but treatment can help slow the progression of the condition and reduce the symptoms. The best way to prevent COPD from quickly getting worse is to stop smoking and avoid further damage to the lungs.

There are also medicines that can help relieve the symptoms of COPD. The type of medicine prescribed will depend on how severe the COPD is and what symptoms the person has. Often, people with COPD have to take a combination of medicines. In addition, many people keep different medicines available in case they have a flare-up, when symptoms are particularly bad.

The person may be prescribed short-acting and/or long-acting inhalers. There are two types of short-acting bronchodilator inhaler: beta-2 agonist inhalers, such as salbutamol and terbutaline and antimuscarinic inhalers, such as ipratropium. Long-acting bronchodilator inhalers: beta-2 agonist inhalers, such as salmeterol and formoterol and/or antimuscarinic inhalers, such as tiotropium, may be prescribed. Steroid inhalers, also called corticosteroid inhalers, work by reducing the inflammation in the airways.

Other treatments include oxygen therapy and in some cases non-invasive ventilation (NIV) may be necessary to control breathing.

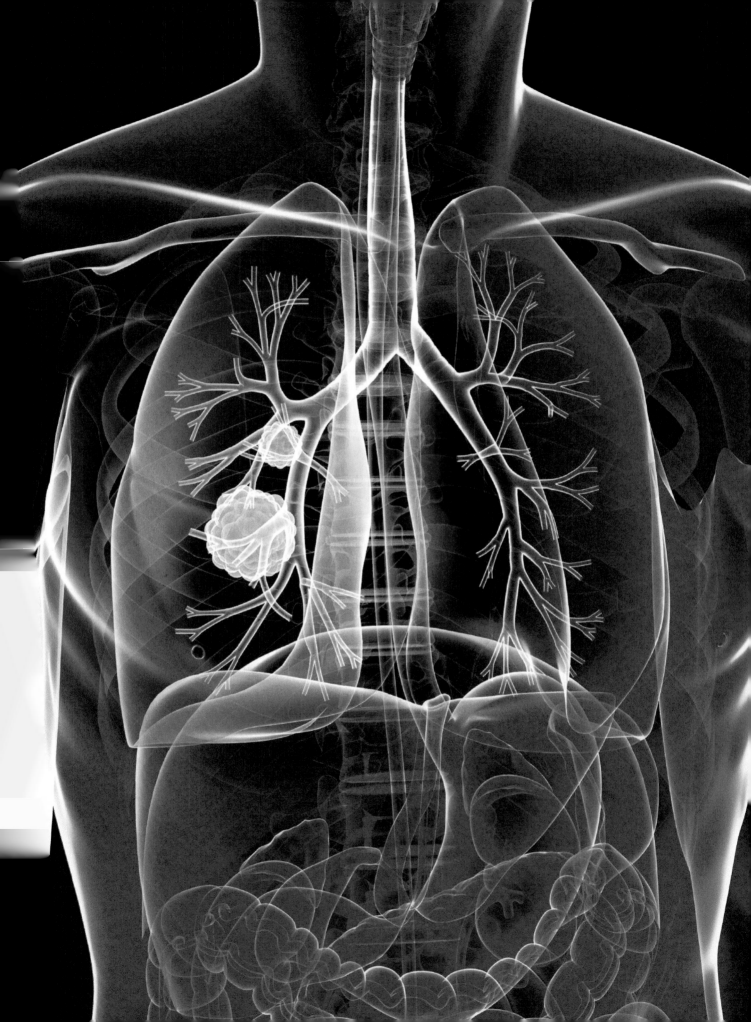

Overview of anatomy and physiology

Peritoneum is the smooth transparent serous membrane that lines the cavity of the abdomen of a mammal and is folded inward over the abdominal and pelvic viscera. The peritoneum is a double-layered serous membrane lining the walls (parietal peritoneum) and organs (visceral peritoneum) of the abdominal cavity (Figure 28.1). There is a potential space between the parietal and visceral layers of the peritoneum that contains a small amount of serous fluid. This space, the peritoneal cavity, is normally sterile.

A small quantity of peritoneal fluid is produced by mesothelial cells. It fills the potential space formed by the two layers of peritoneum and allows the two layers to slide over each other freely. Peritoneal fluid is also produced as a transudate which coats the serosal surface of viscera to facilitate frictionless movement, for example during peristalsis. It is in equilibrium with plasma but doesn't contain high molecular weight molecules like fibrinogen.

The fluid is constantly being produced and resorbed through the large surface area of the peritoneum; for this reason drugs are sometimes administered by intraperitoneal injection. Bacterial toxins are also absorbed readily and can cause inflammation of the peritoneum: peritonitis. Peritoneum secretes a small volume of clear fluid for lubrication. It provides a route for entry of blood, nerve and lymphatics. There is high fibrinolytic activity to protect against the formation of adhesions.

Pathophysiology

Peritonitis results from contamination of the normally sterile peritoneal cavity by infection or a chemical irritant (Figure 28.2). Chemical peritonitis often precedes bacterial peritonitis. Perforation of a peptic ulcer or rupture of the gall bladder releases gastric juices (hydrochloric acid and pepsin) or bile into the peritoneal cavity, causing an acute inflammatory response.

Bacterial peritonitis is usually caused by infection by *Escherichia coli*, *Klebsiella*, *Proteus* or *Pseudomonas* bacteria, which normally inhabit the bowel. Inflammatory and immune defence mechanisms are activated when bacteria enter the peritoneal space. These defences can effectively eliminate small numbers of bacteria, but may be overwhelmed by massive or continued contamination. When this occurs, mast cells release histamine and other vasoactive substances, causing local vasodilation and increased capillary permeability. Polymorphonuclear leukocytes (a type of WBC) infiltrate the peritoneum to phagocytize bacteria and foreign matter. Fibrinogen-rich plasma exudate promotes bacterial destruction and forms fibrin clots to seal off and segregate the bacteria. This process helps limit and localize the infection, allowing host defences to eradicate it. Continued contamination, however, leads to generalized inflammation of the peritoneal cavity. The inflammatory process causes fluid to shift into the peritoneal space (third spacing). Circulating blood volume is depleted, leading to hypovolaemia. Septicaemia, a systemic disease caused by pathogens or their toxins in the blood, may follow.

Peritonitis that develops without an abdominal rupture (spontaneous peritonitis) is usually a complication of liver disease, such as cirrhosis. Advanced cirrhosis causes a large amount of fluid build-up in the abdominal cavity (ascites). That fluid build-up is susceptible to bacterial infection.

Signs and symptoms

Signs and symptoms of peritonitis depend on the severity and extent of the infection, as well as the age and general health of the patient. The patient often presents with evidence of an acute abdomen, an abrupt onset of diffuse, severe abdominal pain. The pain may localize and intensify near the area of infection. Movement may intensify the pain. The entire abdomen is tender, with guarding or rigidity of abdominal muscles. The acute abdomen is often described as board-like. Rebound tenderness may be present over the area of inflammation. Peritoneal inflammation inhibits peristalsis, resulting in a paralytic ileus. Bowel sounds are markedly diminished or absent, and progressive abdominal distention is noted. Pooling of GI secretions may cause nausea and vomiting. Systemic signs of peritonitis include fever, malaise, tachycardia and tachypnoea, restlessness, and possible disorientation. The client may be oliguric (scanty urine output) and show signs of dehydration and shock.

Causes

Most often, peritonitis is caused by an infection that spreads to the peritoneum from another part of the body. This is known as secondary peritonitis. Common causes of secondary peritonitis include perforations from stomach ulcer, burst appendix, Crohn's disease and diverticulitis.

Management

The patient is placed on bed rest due to extreme weakness and shock. The vital signs are monitored regularly. In the early stages they are taken and recorded hourly until the patient is stable. Some patients may be kept nil by mouth due to nausea and vomiting and therefore fluid is administered intravenously.

Many people with peritonitis have problems digesting and processing food, so a feeding tube may be needed. The feeding tube is either passed into the stomach through the nose (nasogastric tube) or surgically placed into the stomach through the abdomen. If these are unsuitable, nutrition may be given directly into one of the veins (parenteral nutrition).

Peritonitis is a serious illness. Early recognition and treatment are important to minimize the risk of complications. The first step in treating peritonitis is determining its underlying cause. Treatment usually involves antibiotics to fight infection and medication for pain.

Surgery

The cause of peritonitis may also need to be surgically treated. For example, if a burst appendix caused the peritonitis, the appendix will need to be removed. Some people develop abscesses (pus-filled swellings) in their peritoneum that need to be drained with a needle. This is carried out using an ultrasound scanner to guide the needle to the abscess.

29 Crohn's disease

Figure 29.1 Areas affected by Crohn's disease

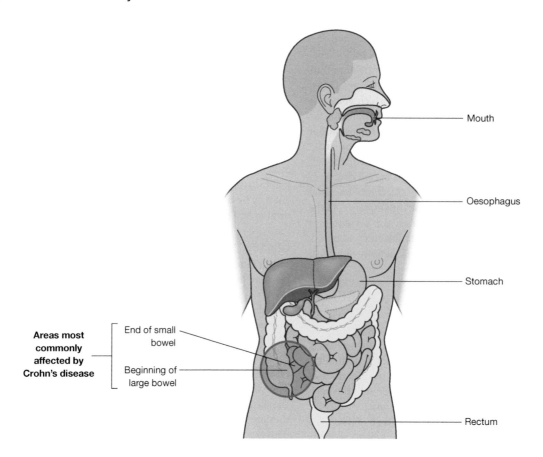

- Mouth
- Oesophagus
- Stomach
- Rectum

Areas most commonly affected by Crohn's disease
- End of small bowel
- Beginning of large bowel

Figure 29.2 Cobblestone appearance of the colon

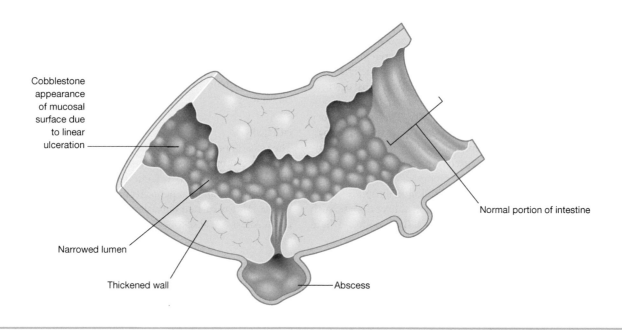

Cobblestone appearance of mucosal surface due to linear ulceration

Normal portion of intestine

Narrowed lumen

Thickened wall

Abscess

Pathophysiology for Nurses at a Glance, First Edition. Muralitharan Nair and Ian Peate. © 2015 John Wiley & Sons, Ltd. Published 2015 by John Wiley & Sons, Ltd.
Companion website: www.ataglanceseries.com/nursing/pathophysiology

Overview of anatomy and physiology

Crohn's disease is a long-term condition that causes inflammation of the lining of the digestive system. Any part of the gut can be affected (Figure 29.1). However, the most common site for the disease to start is the last part of the small intestine (the ileum).

The gut (gastrointestinal tract) is the long tube that starts at the mouth and ends at the anus. When we eat, food passes down the oesophagus (gullet), into the stomach and then into the small intestine.

The small intestine has three sections: the duodenum, jejunum and ileum. The small intestine is where food is digested and absorbed into the bloodstream. The structure of the gut then changes to become the large intestine (colon and rectum, sometimes called the large bowel).

The colon absorbs water, and contains food that has not been digested, such as fibre. This is passed into the last part of the large intestine, where it is stored as faeces. Faeces (stools) are then passed out of the anus into the toilet.

Pathophysiology

A patch of inflammation may be small, or spread quite a distance along part of the gut. Several patches of inflammation may develop along the gut, with normal sections of gut in between. In about three in ten cases, the inflammation occurs just in the small intestine. In about two in ten cases the inflammation occurs just in the colon. In a number of cases, the inflammation occurs in different places in the gut.

The lumen of the affected bowel assumes a 'cobblestone' appearance as fissures and ulcers surround islands of intact mucosa over oedematous submucosa (Figure 29.2). The inflammatory lesions of Crohn's disease are not continuous; rather, they often occur as 'skip' lesions, with intervening areas of normal-appearing bowel. Some evidence suggests that despite its normal appearance, the entire bowel is affected by this disorder.

Depending on the severity and extent of the disease, malabsorption and malnutrition may develop as the ulcers prevent absorption of nutrients. When the jejunum and ileum are affected, the absorption of multiple nutrients may be impaired, including carbohydrates, proteins, fats, vitamins and folate. Disease in the terminal ileum can lead to vitamin B_{12} malabsorption and bile salt reabsorption. The ulcerations can also lead to protein loss and chronic, slow blood loss, with consequent anaemia.

Risk factors

The exact cause of Crohn's disease is unknown. However, some possible factors include: some genetic factors; the inflammation may be caused by a problem with the immune system (the body's defence against infection and illness) that causes it to attack healthy bacteria in the gut; smokers with Crohn's disease usually have more severe symptoms than non-smokers; previous infection may trigger an abnormal response from the immune system; and Crohn's disease is most common in westernized countries, such as the UK, and least common in poorer parts of the world, such as Africa.

Signs and symptoms

The symptoms of Crohn's vary depending on which part of the digestive system is inflamed. Some of the common symptoms include diarrhoea, abdominal pain, fatigue, weight loss, fever, malaise and anaemia. Stools are liquid or semi-formed and do not contain blood. There may be long periods of mild symptoms followed by periods where the symptoms are particularly troublesome.

Management

Diet

Eating a healthy, balanced diet is important for everyone, including in Crohn's disease. Patients may find that they are sensitive to certain foods which can make the symptoms worse. If this happens, then removing these foods from the diet can help. Always get advice from a dietitian before making any changes to the diet. During a flare-up, a liquid diet made up of simple forms of protein, carbohydrates and fats may help to ease the symptoms.

Medicines

Some of the medication used in the treatment of Crohn's disease includes corticosteroids (such as hydrocortisone, beclometasone and budesonide). These are very effective but are usually used for a short time during a flare-up because they can cause weight gain and side effects such as diabetes and osteoporosis. Immunosuppressants may also be used to suppress the immune system (such as azathioprine, mercaptopurine and methotrexate), and antibiotics to reduce the risk of infection.

Surgery

Surgery is often required when the symptoms of Crohn's disease cannot be controlled using medication alone. An estimated 80% of people with Crohn's disease do require surgery at some point in their life. Surgery cannot cure Crohn's disease but it can provide long periods of remission, often lasting several years. During surgery, the inflamed section of the digestive system is removed and the remaining part is reattached.

Complications

Certain complications of Crohn's disease (e.g. intestinal obstruction, abscess and fistula) are so common that they are considered part of the disease process. For many clients, the disease initially presents with one of these complications. Intestinal obstruction is a common complication caused by repeated inflammation and scarring of the bowel that leads to fibrosis and stricture. Obstruction of the bowel lumen causes abdominal distention, cramping pain, and nausea and vomiting.

Perforation of the bowel is uncommon, but can lead to generalized peritonitis. Massive haemorrhage also is an uncommon complication of Crohn's disease. Long-standing Crohn's disease increases the risk of cancer of the small intestine or colon by 5–6 times.

30 Peptic ulcer

Figure 30.1 Digestive system

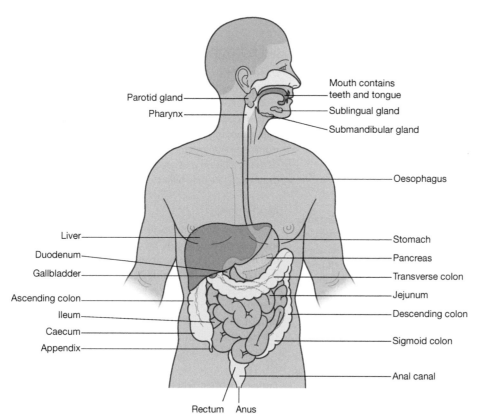

Parotid gland
Pharynx
Mouth contains teeth and tongue
Sublingual gland
Submandibular gland
Oesophagus
Liver
Duodenum
Gallbladder
Ascending colon
Ileum
Caecum
Appendix
Stomach
Pancreas
Transverse colon
Jejunum
Descending colon
Sigmoid colon
Anal canal
Rectum   Anus

Source:
Peate, Wild & Nair, *Nursing Practice: Knowledge and Care,* 2014

Figure 30.2 Peptic (gastric) ulcer

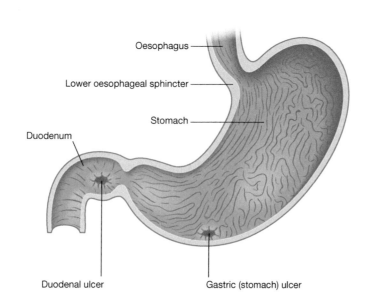

Oesophagus
Lower oesophageal sphincter
Stomach
Duodenum
Duodenal ulcer
Gastric (stomach) ulcer

Figure 30.3 Diagram of a *H. Pylori*

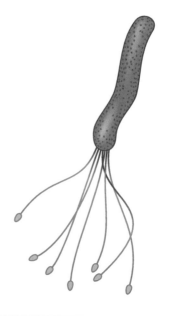

Pathophysiology for Nurses at a Glance, First Edition. Muralitharan Nair and Ian Peate. © 2015 John Wiley & Sons, Ltd. Published 2015 by John Wiley & Sons, Ltd.
Companion website: www.ataglanceseries.com/nursing/pathophysiology

Overview of anatomy and physiology

Food passes down the oesophagus (gullet) into the stomach (Figure 30.1). The stomach makes acid which is not essential, but helps to digest food. After being mixed in the stomach, food passes into the duodenum (the first part of the small intestine). In the duodenum and the rest of the small intestine, food mixes with enzymes (chemicals). The enzymes come from the pancreas and from cells lining the intestine. The enzymes break down (digest) the food which is absorbed into the body.

The stomach may be divided into seven major sections. The cardia is a 1–2 cm segment distal to the oesophagogastric junction. The fundus refers to the superior portion of the stomach that lies above an imaginary horizontal plane that passes through the oesophagogastric junction. The antrum is the smaller distal a quarter to a third of the stomach. The narrow 1–2 cm channel that connects the stomach and duodenum is the pylorus. The lesser curve refers to the medial shorter border of the stomach, whereas the opposite surface is the greater curve.

Pathophysiology

Ulcers are caused when there is an imbalance between the digestive juices produced by the stomach and the various factors that protect the lining of the stomach. Symptoms of ulcers may include bleeding. On rare occasions, an ulcer may completely erode the stomach wall.

Mucus lines the digestive tract and acts as a barrier against the acidic gastric secretions. Too little mucus production coupled with too much acid production will leave the digestive tract vulnerable to acid erosion and ulceration. Erosion of the mucosal lining may result in the formation of a fistula. The fistula would allow the acidic gastric contents to leak out into the peritoneum, resulting in peritonitis. Stress, caffeine, cigarette smoking and alcohol consumption increase acid production. Medications such as NSAIDs and aspirin inhibit prostaglandins which protects mucosal lining.

Causes

A peptic ulcer is an area of damage to the inner lining (the mucosa) of the stomach or the upper part of the intestine (duodenum) (Figure 30.2). A bacterium, *Helicobacter pylori*, is the main cause of ulcers in this area. *H. pylori* bacterial (Figure 30.3) infection leads to death of the mucosal epithelial cells of the stomach and duodenum. The bacteria release toxins and enzymes that reduce the efficiency of mucous in protecting the mucosal lining of the gastrointestinal tract. In response to the bacterial infection, the body initiates an inflammatory response which results in further destruction of the mucosal lining and ulceration.

However, the ulcer can be caused by the use of painkillers called non-steroidal anti-inflammatory drugs (NSAIDs), such as aspirin, naproxen (Aleve, Anaprox, Naprosyn and others), ibuprofen (Motrin, Advil, Midol and others), and many others available by prescription. Even safety-coated aspirin and aspirin in powdered form can frequently cause ulcers.

Other causes include excess acid production from gastrinomas, tumours of the acid producing cells of the stomach that increase acid output (seen in Zollinger-Ellison syndrome). Smoking, stress, excessive consumption of caffeine and familial history have also been included as risk factors for peptic ulcer.

Signs and symptoms

Some patients with peptic ulcer have no symptoms. However, for some the possible symptoms include epigastric pain, heart burn, poor appetite, burping and feeling bloated. This pain is often described as burning or gnawing and may extend to the back. It usually comes on after eating – often 1–2 hours after a meal – and may come and go for several days or weeks.

Management

Once peptic ulcer has been diagnosed, the nurse should help the patient identify any lifestyle factors which may be associated with peptic ulcers, such as stress, heavy alcohol consumption, smoking or drinking a lot of coffee. Once identified, the nurse and patient can discuss ways of reducing the risks.

Nearly all duodenal ulcers are caused by infection with *H. pylori*. Therefore, a main part of the treatment is to clear this infection. If this infection is not cleared, the ulcer is likely to return once acid-suppressing medication is stopped. Two antibiotics are needed. In addition, an acid-suppressing medicine is needed to reduce the acid in the stomach. This is needed to allow the antibiotics to work well. The patient may need to take this combination therapy (sometimes called triple therapy) for a week.

Medication

A 4–8 week course of a medicine that greatly reduces the amount of acid that the stomach makes is usually advised. The most commonly used medicine is a proton pump inhibitor (PPI). This is a class (group) of medicines that work on the cells that line the stomach, reducing the production of acid. They include: esomeprazole, lansoprazole, omeprazole, pantoprazole and rabeprazole, and come in various brand names. Sometimes another class of medicines called H2 blockers is used. They are also called histamine H2-receptor antagonists, but are commonly called H2 blockers. H2 blockers work in a different way on the cells that line the stomach, reducing the production of acid. They include: cimetidine, famotidine, nizatidine and ranitidine, and come in various brand names. As the amount of acid is greatly reduced, the ulcer usually heals.

Diet

Dietary advice should be offered to the patient. Small regular meals are encouraged, approximately five small meals per day to prevent hunger pain. Spicy food should be avoided as it may cause irritation on the mucosal membrane of the stomach, resulting in inflammation and epigastric pain.

31 Ulcerative colitis

Figure 31.1 Diagram of the colon affected by ulcerative colitis

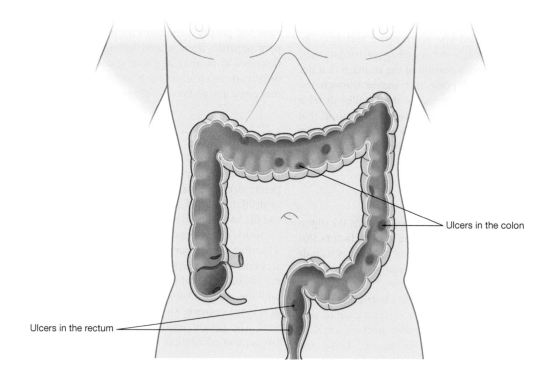

Ulcers in the colon

Ulcers in the rectum

Figure 31.2 Diagram showing colonoscopy procedure

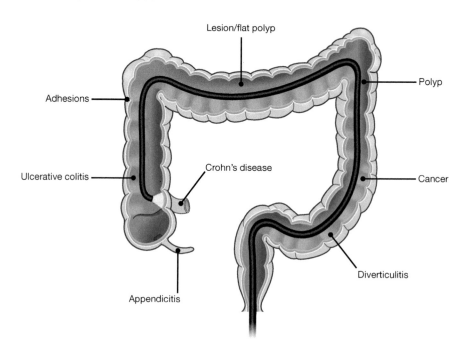

Lesion/flat polyp

Adhesions

Polyp

Ulcerative colitis

Crohn's disease

Cancer

Appendicitis

Diverticulitis

Pathophysiology for Nurses at a Glance, First Edition. Muralitharan Nair and Ian Peate. © 2015 John Wiley & Sons, Ltd. Published 2015 by John Wiley & Sons, Ltd.
Companion website: www.ataglanceseries.com/nursing/pathophysiology

Overview of anatomy and physiology

Ulcerative colitis (UC) is a disease where inflammation develops in the colon and the rectum (the large intestine) (Figure 31.1). Ulcerative colitis is one of the two main inflammatory bowel diseases; the other being Crohn's disease. Sometimes, ulcerative colitis only affects the rectum – this is called proctitis and is a less severe condition.

Ulcerative colitis is found worldwide, but is most common in the USA, England and northern Europe. It is especially common in people of Jewish descent. Ulcerative colitis is rarely seen in Eastern Europe, Asia and South America, and is rare in the black population. For unknown reasons, an increased frequency of this condition has been observed recently in developing nations. For an overview of the GI tract refer to Chapter 29.

Pathophysiology

What is ulcerative colitis?

'Colitis' means inflammation of the colon. 'Ulcerative' means that ulcers tend to develop, often in places where there is inflammation. An ulcer occurs when the lining of the gut is damaged and the underlying tissue is exposed. Inside the gastrointestinal tract (gut), an ulcer looks like a small, red crater on the inside lining. Ulcers that occur in UC develop in the large intestine and have a tendency to bleed.

Inflammatory processes occur in the mucosa and the submucosa of the rectum (proctitis) and spread along the colon. The inflammation may involve the entire colon up to the junction of the ileocaecal valve. The inflammation and mucosal destruction leads to swelling, oedema and bleeding and as the disease progresses ulceration develops. Mucosal destruction also leads to an increase in the urge to defaecate, with patients having to go to the toilet over ten times per day. Some patients will have iron deficiency anaemia. The ulceration spreads through the submucosa, causing necrosis and sloughing of the mucous membrane. In later stages of the disease, the walls of the colon thicken and become fibrous. This leads to a narrowing of the lumen of the large intestine, which can lead to intestinal obstruction. Loss of normal large intestine function can lead to complications such as dehydration, and electrolyte imbalance may develop. Abdominal cramping and pain are associated with these attacks.

How is ulcerative colitis diagnosed?

The usual test is for a doctor to look inside the colon and the rectum (the large intestine) by passing a special telescope up through the back passage (anus) into the rectum and colon. These are a short sigmoidoscope or a longer flexible colonoscope (Figure 31.2). The appearance of the inside lining of the rectum and colon may suggest UC. Small samples (biopsies) are taken from the lining of the rectum and colon and looked at under the microscope. The typical pattern of the cells seen with the microscope may confirm the diagnosis. Also, various blood tests are usually done to check for anaemia and to assess general well-being.

Special X-ray tests, such as a barium enema, are not often done these days, as the above tests are used to confirm the diagnosis and assess the disease severity.

A stool sample (sample of faeces) is commonly done during each flare-up and sent to the laboratory to test for bacteria and other infecting germs. Although no germ has been proven initially to cause UC, infection with various known germs can trigger a flare-up of symptoms. If a germ is found, then treatment of this may be needed in addition to any other treatment for a flare-up.

Signs and symptoms

These can vary depending on how much of the colon is affected and the level of inflammation. Some of the symptoms reported include abdominal pain, diarrhoea with blood and/or mucous, anaemia, weight loss and poor appetite. There may be symptoms of systemic upset, including malaise, fever and symptoms of extra-intestinal (joint, cutaneous and eye) manifestations.

Depending on disease severity, the patient may be clearly unwell, pale, febrile and dehydrated. He or she may have a tachycardia and hypotension.

Management

The patient with ulcerative colitis may need psychological support and counselling. Depression may be a result of the debilitating disease and the person may feel isolated. As a result of diarrhoea and bowel habits, the patient may be reluctant to engage in social activity and feel a burden to their family. The patient should be allowed to express their anxieties and worries about the disease.

It is easy to become dehydrated with ulcerative colitis, as a lot of fluid may be lost through diarrhoea. Water is the best source of fluids. Caffeine and alcohol should be avoided as these will make the diarrhoea worse; and fizzy drinks tend to cause gas. Advise the patient to keep a food diary to identify food that he/she can tolerate and the ones that make the symptoms worse. By keeping a record of what and when they eat, they should be able to eliminate problem foods from the diet.

Fluid intake and output must be monitored, ensure that the patient is not dehydrated. Dehydration may be a possibility as a result of the diarrhoea. Electrolyte balance needs to be monitored daily as a result of the loss of electrolytes such as sodium and potassium in the vomit and diarrhoea.

Living with ulcerative colitis can be frustrating and isolating. Talking to others with the condition can be of great benefit. Encourage the patient to see their practice nurse when symptoms get worse or when they are worried.

32 Bowel cancer

Figure 32.1 The large bowel (colon)

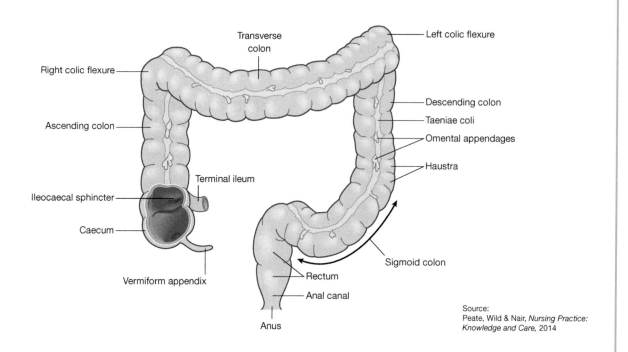

Transverse colon

Right colic flexure

Left colic flexure

Ascending colon

Descending colon

Taeniae coli

Omental appendages

Haustra

Terminal ileum

Ileocaecal sphincter

Caecum

Vermiform appendix

Sigmoid colon

Rectum

Anal canal

Anus

Source:
Peate, Wild & Nair, *Nursing Practice:
Knowledge and Care*, 2014

Figure 32.2 Spread of cancer cells into the bloodstream and lymphatic system

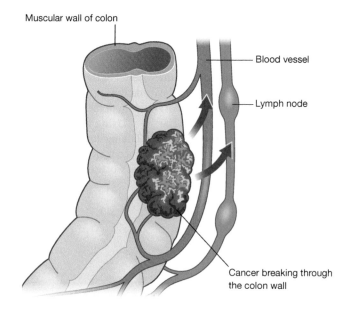

Muscular wall of colon

Blood vessel

Lymph node

Cancer breaking through
the colon wall

Overview of anatomy and physiology

Bowel cancer (also known as colorectal cancer) affects the lower part of the digestive system – the large bowel and the rectum. It affects men and women equally, and is the third most common type of cancer in men and the second most common in women. One in twenty people in the UK will develop bowel cancer in their lifetime.

The colon and rectum are parts of the gastrointestinal tract. The gut starts at the mouth and ends at the anus. When we eat or drink, the food and liquid travel down the oesophagus into the stomach. The stomach churns up the food and then passes it into the small intestine.

The small intestine (sometimes called the small bowel) is several metres long and is where food is digested and absorbed. Undigested food, water and waste products are then passed into the large intestine (sometimes called the large bowel). The main part of the large intestine is called the colon, which is about 150 cm long. This is split into four sections: the ascending, transverse, descending and sigmoid colon (Figure 32.1). Some water and salts are absorbed into the body from the colon. The colon leads into the rectum (back passage), which is about 15 cm long. The rectum stores faeces (stools) before they are passed out from the anus.

Pathophysiology
What is cancer?

Cancer is a disease of the cells in the body. The body is made up of millions of tiny cells. There are many different types of cell in the body, and there are many different types of cancer which arise from different types of cell. What all types of cancer have in common is that the cancer cells are abnormal and multiply out of control.

A malignant tumour is a lump or growth of tissue made up from cancer cells which continue to multiply. Malignant tumours invade into nearby tissues and organs, which can cause damage. Malignant tumours may also spread to other parts of the body. This happens if some cells break off from the primary tumour and are carried in the bloodstream or lymph channels to other parts of the body. These small groups of cells may then multiply to form secondary tumours (metastases) in one or more parts of the body. These secondary tumours may then grow, invade and damage nearby tissues and can spread again.

Some cancers are more serious than others, some are more easily treated than others (particularly if diagnosed at an early stage), some have a better prognosis than others.

What is bowel cancer?

Bowel cancer is a cancer of the colon or rectum. It is sometimes called bowel cancer or cancer of the large intestine. It is one of the most common cancers in the UK. Bowel cancer can affect any part of the colon or rectum. However, it most commonly develops in the lower part of the descending colon, the sigmoid colon or rectum. Nearly all colorectal cancers are adenocarcinomas that begin as adenomatous polyps.

Bowel cancer usually develops from a polyp which has formed on the lining of the colon or rectum. Sometimes bowel cancer begins from a cell within the lining of the colon or rectum which becomes cancerous. Some rare types of cancer arise from various other cells in the wall of the colon or rectum, for example carcinoid, lymphoma and sarcomas.

As the cancer cells multiply they form a tumour. The tumour invades deeper into the wall of the colon or rectum. Some cells may break off into the lymph channels or bloodstream (Figure 32.2). The cancer may then metastasize to lymph nodes nearby or to other areas of the body – most commonly, the liver and lungs.

Signs and symptoms

When a colorectal cancer first develops and is small it usually causes no symptoms. As it grows, the symptoms that develop can vary, depending on the site of the tumour. Some of the symptoms include: bleeding, passing mucus with the stool, abdominal pain, a feeling of not fully emptying the rectum after passing faeces and change in bowel habits. If the cancer becomes very large, it can cause a blockage (obstruction) of the colon. This causes severe abdominal pain and other symptoms such as vomiting.

Management

Surgical resection of the tumour, adjacent colon and regional lymph nodes is the treatment of choice for colorectal cancer. Options for surgical treatment vary, from destruction of the tumour by laser photocoagulation performed during endoscopy, to abdominoperineal resection with permanent colostomy. When possible, the anal sphincter is preserved and colostomy avoided.

Most clients with colorectal cancer undergo surgical resection of the colon, with anastomosis of remaining bowel as a curative procedure. The distribution of regional lymph nodes determines the extent of resection because these may contain metastatic lesions. Most tumours of the ascending, transverse, descending and sigmoid colon can be resected.

Tumours of the rectum are usually treated with an abdominoperineal resection in which the sigmoid colon, rectum and anus are removed through both abdominal and perineal incisions. A permanent sigmoid colostomy is performed to provide for elimination of faeces.

Radiotherapy may be used to kill cancer cells. Doctors don't often use it to treat cancer in the colon. But they often use it to treat cancer that started in the rectum. Usually, this treatment is given at the same time as 5FU (fluorouracil) chemotherapy. The chemotherapy makes the cancer cells more sensitive to radiation.

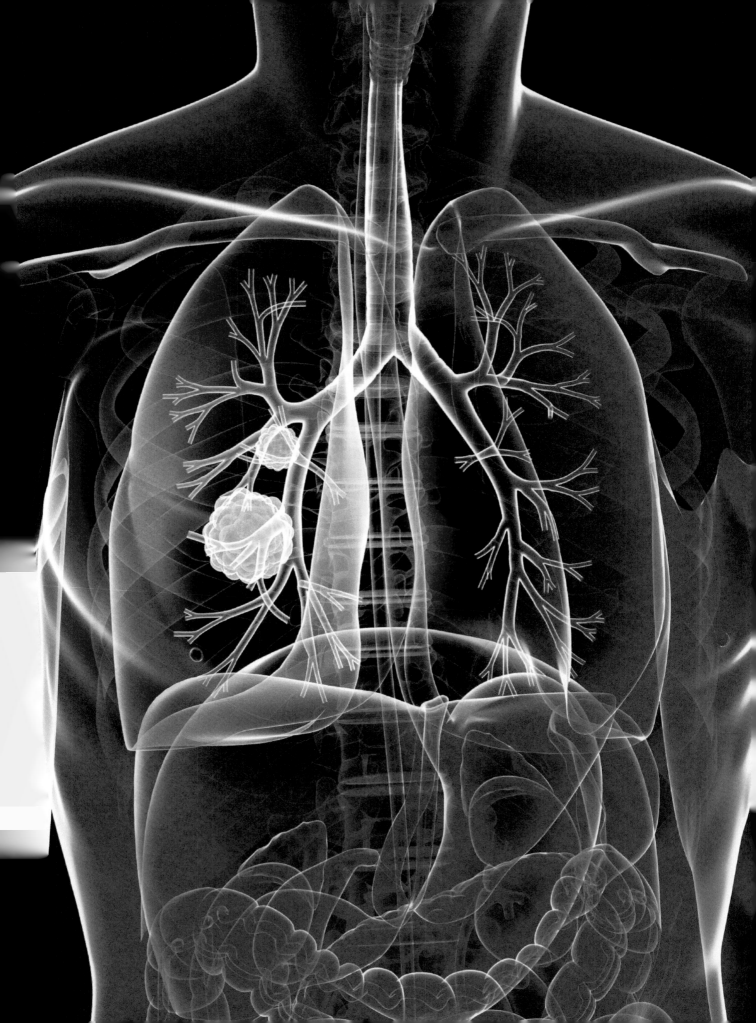

Overview of anatomy and physiology

The gall bladder is a hollow system that sits just beneath the liver. In adults, the gall bladder measures approximately 8 cm in length and 4 cm in diameter when fully distended. It is divided into three sections: fundus, body and neck (Figure 34.1).

Bile production is the liver's primary digestive function. Bile is a greenish, watery solution containing bile salts, cholesterol, bilirubin, electrolytes, water and phospholipids. These substances are necessary to emulsify and promote the absorption of fats. Liver cells make 700–1200 mL of bile daily. When bile is not needed for digestion, the sphincter of Oddi (Figure 34.1) (located at the point at which bile enters the duodenum) is closed, and the bile backs up the cystic duct into the gall bladder for storage.

Bile is concentrated and stored in the gall bladder, a small sac cupped in the inferior surface of the liver. When food containing fats enters the duodenum, hormones stimulate the gall bladder to secrete bile into the cystic duct. The cystic duct joins the hepatic duct to form the common bile duct, from which bile enters into the duodenum.

Pathophysiology

Cholecystitis is inflammation (swelling) of the gall bladder. It is usually caused by a gallstone that becomes trapped in one of the ducts or openings of the gall bladder (Figure 34.2). Acute cholecystitis usually follows obstruction of the cystic duct by a stone. Chronic cholecystitis may result from repeated bouts of acute cholecystitis or from persistent irritation of the gall bladder wall by stones.

Gallstones are small stones, usually made of cholesterol, that form in the gall bladder. In most cases they do not cause any symptoms. Gallstones form when several factors interact: abnormal bile composition, biliary stasis and inflammation of the gall bladder. Most gallstones (80%) consist primarily of cholesterol; the rest contain a mixture of bile components. Excess cholesterol in bile is associated with obesity, a high-calorie, high-cholesterol diet and drugs that lower serum cholesterol levels. When bile is supersaturated with cholesterol, it can precipitate out to form stones. Biliary stasis, or slowed emptying of the gall bladder, contributes to cholelithiasis. Stones do not form when the gall bladder empties completely in response to hormonal stimulation. Slowed or incomplete emptying allows cholesterol to concentrate and increases the risk of stone formation. Finally, inflammation of the gall bladder allows excess water and bile salt reabsorption, increasing the risk for lithiasis.

How is cholecystitis diagnosed?

An ultrasound scan is commonly done to clarify the diagnosis. This is a painless test which uses sound waves to scan the abdomen. An ultrasound scan can usually detect gallstones, and also whether the wall of the gall bladder is thickened (as occurs with cholecystitis). If the diagnosis is in doubt then other more detailed scans may be done.

Blood test: a higher than normal white blood cell count may indicate that there is an infection. Higher levels of bilirubin, alkaline phosphatase and serum aninotransferase may also help the doctor make a diagnosis.

Signs and symptoms

Cholecystitis usually presents as a pain in the right upper quadrant or epigastric region. The gall bladder may be tender and distended. Symptomatically it differs from biliary colic by the presence of an inflammatory component (fever, increased white cell count). Pain is initially intermittent, but later usually presents as constant and severe. The pain may be referred pain that is felt in the right scapula rather than the right upper quadrant or epigastric region (Boas' sign). It may also correlate with eating greasy, fatty or fried foods. Diarrhoea, vomiting and nausea are common. The Murphy sign is specific, but not sensitive for cholecystitis.

Management

The patient with gall bladder disorder is very ill and may be in shock as a result of severe nausea and vomiting. The priority is to admit the patient and administer appropriate analgesia, keep him/her nil by mouth due to nausea and vomiting, monitor vital signs hourly and observe signs and symptoms of shock until the condition stabilizes; give fluids by intravenous infusion to prevent dehydration and monitor urea and electrolyte levels.

Surgery

Cholecystectomy is carried out either using a laparoscopic or through an open cholecystectomy. Unless the patient requires an open cholecystectomy, the preferred surgical procedure is laparoscopic cholecystectomy for gall bladder disorders. It is called keyhole surgery as only small cuts are needed in the abdomen, with small scars remaining afterwards. The recovery of the patient following this procedure is much quicker than when open surgery is carried out.

Alternative treatment

Extracorporeal shockwave lithotripsy (ECSL): shock waves are used to break up or dissolve the stones so that they can be passed via the GI tract.

Oral dissolution therapy: gallstones that are made of cholesterol can sometimes be treated using a medication called ursodeoxycholic acid, which slowly dissolves gallstones. Ursodeoxycholic acid is also sometimes prescribed as a precaution against gallstones if it is thought that the patient has a high risk of developing gallstones.

Contact dissolution therapy: drugs to dissolve the stones are introduced into the gall bladder via a tube through the skin.

Diet: after a cholecystectomy there is no need to follow a low fat diet. A low fat diet may result in weight loss. However, due to the role that cholesterol appears to play in the formation of gallstones, it is recommended to avoid eating fatty foods that have a high cholesterol content.

35 Pancreatitis

Figure 35.1 Diagram of a pancreas

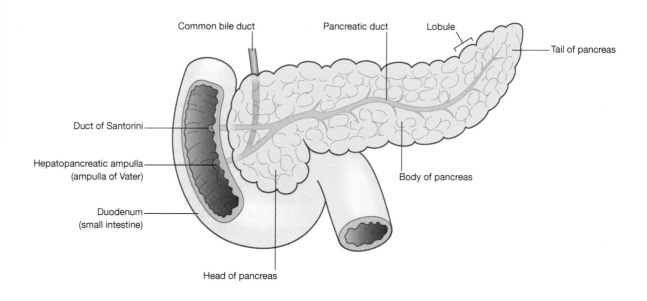

Common bile duct

Pancreatic duct

Lobule

Tail of pancreas

Duct of Santorini

Hepatopancreatic ampulla
(ampulla of Vater)

Duodenum
(small intestine)

Body of pancreas

Head of pancreas

Figure 35.2 Diagram showing inflamed pancreas due to gallstone blocking the duct

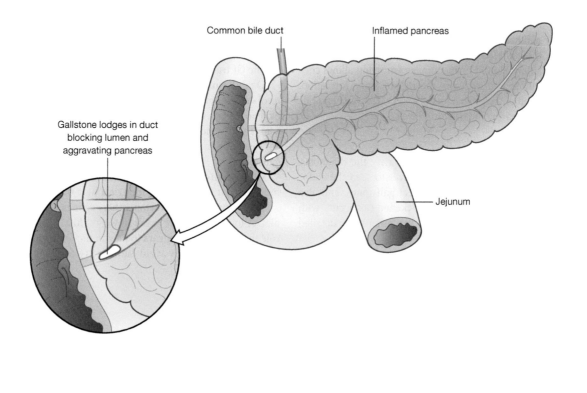

Common bile duct

Inflamed pancreas

Gallstone lodges in duct
blocking lumen and
aggravating pancreas

Jejunum

Pathophysiology for Nurses at a Glance, First Edition. Muralitharan Nair and Ian Peate. © 2015 John Wiley & Sons, Ltd. Published 2015 by John Wiley & Sons, Ltd.
Companion website: www.ataglanceseries.com/nursing/pathophysiology

Overview of anatomy and physiology

The pancreas is in the upper half of the abdomen, level with the V-shape where the ribs meet at the front. It lies behind the stomach and just in front of the backbone. It is about 15 cm long and is shaped like a tadpole. The large rounded section is called the head of the pancreas and lies next to the first part of the small bowel (the duodenum). The middle part is known as the body of the pancreas. The narrow part is called the tail of the pancreas (Figure 35.1).

The pancreas has two main functions: to make digestive enzymes which help us to digest food and to make hormones which regulate our metabolism. Enzymes are special chemicals which help to speed up body's processes. Hormones are chemicals which can be released into the bloodstream. They act as messengers, affecting cells and tissues in distant parts of the body.

Pancreatic juices travel through small tubes (ducts) in the pancreas into a larger duct called the pancreatic duct. This joins with the bile duct, which carries bile from the liver and gall bladder, before opening into the duodenum. The pancreatic juices flow along the pancreatic duct into the duodenum where they help to digest food.

Pathophysiology

Acute pancreatitis

In acute pancreatitis the inflammation develops quickly (Figure 35.2), over a few days or so. It often goes away completely and leaves no permanent damage. Sometimes it is serious. Some of the causes include:

Gallstones: the most common cause in the UK. A gallstone can pass through the bile duct and out into part of the gut just after the stomach (the duodenum). This usually does not cause a problem. However, in some people a gallstone gets stuck in the bile duct or where the bile duct and pancreatic duct open into the duodenum. This can affect the enzymes in the pancreatic duct (or even block them completely) and trigger a pancreatitis.

Alcohol: is the other common cause. How alcohol actually triggers the inflammation in the pancreas is not clear. Symptoms typically begin about 6–12 hours after a heavy drinking session. In some people, pancreatitis can develop even after a small amount of alcohol. In these people, a 'sensitivity' to alcohol develops in their pancreas.

Autoimmune: this is where the body's own immune system attacks the pancreas. This can be associated with other autoimmune diseases, for example Sjögren's syndrome and primary biliary cirrhosis.

Chronic pancreatitis

Chronic pancreatitis occurs when the inflammation is persistent. The inflammation tends to be less intense than acute pancreatitis, but as it is ongoing it can cause scarring and damage. About 4 in 100 people across the world at any one time have chronic pancreatitis. It is not known exactly how many people in the UK have this condition, but it is thought to have increased considerably over the years. It is more common in men than in women. Some causes include:

Alcohol: the common cause (about seven in ten cases). Men aged 40–50 are the most common group of people affected. In most cases the person has been drinking heavily for ten years or more before symptoms first begin.

Genetic: there are some rare genetic conditions which can lead to chronic pancreatitis developing. Cystic fibrosis can be one cause. 'Genetic' means that someone is born with it and it is passed on through families through special codes inside cells, called genes.

Autoimmune: this is where someone's own immune system attacks the pancreas. This can be associated with other autoimmune diseases. For example, Sjögren's syndrome and primary biliary cirrhosis.

Signs and symptoms

The pain usually develops in the middle or on the left side of the abdomen and can sometimes travel along the back. Some people may experience a constant mild to moderate pain in their abdomen in between episodes of severe pain. This pattern of symptoms is most common in people who continue to drink alcohol after being diagnosed with chronic pancreatitis.

Additional symptoms can occur when the pancreas loses its ability to produce digestive juices, which help break down food in the digestive system. The pancreas usually only loses these functions many years after the original symptoms started. Other symptoms include nausea and vomiting, jaundice and loss of appetite. Diabetes is also a common symptom, which affects over half of all patients with long-standing chronic pancreatitis.

Management

The treatment of acute pancreatitis is largely supportive. Narcotic analgesics such as morphine are used to control pain. Antibiotics are often prescribed to prevent or treat infection.

Oral food and fluids are withheld during acute episodes of pancreatitis to reduce pancreatic secretions and promote rest of the organ. A nasogastric tube may be inserted and connected to suction. Intravenous fluids are administered to maintain vascular volume, and total parenteral nutrition (TPN) is initiated. Oral food and fluids are begun once the serum amylase levels have returned to normal, bowel sounds are present, and pain disappears. A low-fat diet is ordered, and alcohol intake is strictly prohibited.

Clients with chronic pancreatitis may need to remain on pancreatic enzyme supplements for life. H_2 blockers, such as cimetidine (Tagamet) and ranitidine (Zantac), and proton-pump inhibitors, such as omeprazole (Prilosec) may be given to neutralize or decrease gastric secretions.

Remind family and visitors to avoid bringing food into the client's room. The sight or smell of food may stimulate secretory activity of the pancreas through the cephalic phase of digestion.

36 Liver cancer

Figure 36.1 The liver segments

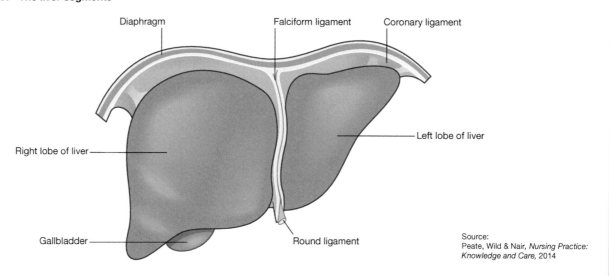

Diaphragm
Falciform ligament
Coronary ligament
Left lobe of liver
Right lobe of liver
Gallbladder
Round ligament

Source:
Peate, Wild & Nair, *Nursing Practice: Knowledge and Care*, 2014

Figure 36.2 Cirrhosis of the liver

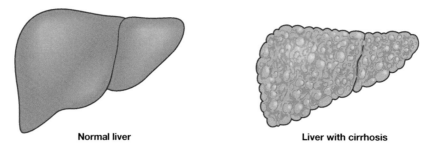

Normal liver

Liver with cirrhosis

Figure 36.3 Drainage of ascites from the abdomen

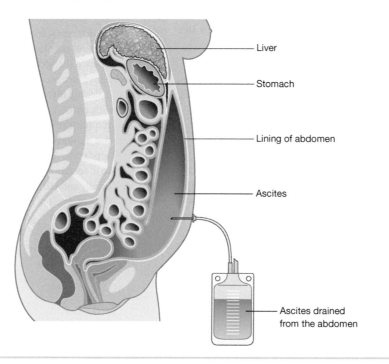

Liver
Stomach
Lining of abdomen
Ascites
Ascites drained
from the abdomen

Overview of anatomy and physiology

The liver is the second largest organ in the body after the skin. It is found below the right lung and is protected by the lower ribs on that side. The liver is divided into two main lobes, the larger right lobe and two smaller lobes. The two main lobes are further divided into eight segments.

The liver is one of the most complex organs in the human body. It has more than 500 functions. Some of the liver's most important functions include: digesting proteins and fats, removing toxins (poisons) from the body, helping to control blood clotting (thickening) and releasing bile, a liquid that breaks down fats and aids digestion.

Pathophysiology

Primary liver cancer is relatively rare in the UK, but it is increasing. Worldwide, it is the sixth most common cancer. The highest rates are in Eastern Asia.

About 80–90% of primary hepatic cancers arise from the liver's parenchymal cells (hepatocellular carcinoma); the remainder form in the bile ducts (cholangiocarcinoma). Regardless of the origin, the progress of the disease is similar. Most primary liver cancer is related to alcoholic cirrhosis, HBV or HCV.

Tumours may be limited to one specific area, may occur as nodules throughout the liver, or may develop as surface infiltrates. The tumour interferes with normal hepatic function, leading to biliary obstruction and jaundice, portal hypertension and metabolic disruptions (hypoalbuminaemia, hypoglycaemia and bleeding disorders). It may also secrete bile products and produce hormones (paraneoplastic syndrome) that may lead to polycythaemia, hypoglycaemia, and hypercalcaemia. Tumours usually grow rapidly and metastasize early.

Risk factors

As people get older, their risk of developing hepatocellular carcinoma (HCC) increases – 70% are in people over 65. Cirrhosis is scarring throughout the liver, which can be due to a variety of causes. These include chronic infection (see below), heavy alcohol drinking over a long period of time, obesity that causes chronic fatty liver disease and a few rare conditions, such as haemochromatosis (a genetic condition) and primary biliary cirrhosis.

Liver cirrhosis (Figure 36.2) increases the risk of developing HCC. The risk varies depending on the cause of the cirrhosis. However, only a small number of people with liver cirrhosis will develop primary liver cancer.

Long-term infection with either the hepatitis B or hepatitis C virus can lead to liver cancer and can cause cirrhosis, which increases the risk of HCC. People with hepatitis B or C should avoid excessive amounts of alcohol, as this can further increase their risk of developing primary liver cancer.

Smoking increases the risk of liver cancer. Researchers estimate that almost a quarter of liver cancers in the UK are caused by smoking. In smokers who also have hepatitis C or hepatitis B virus infection the risk is increased further. Smokers who drink large amounts of alcohol may have a risk that is up to ten times higher than people who don't smoke or drink.

Signs and symptoms

Jaundice can occur if the liver isn't working properly because of cancer or an underlying disease, such as cirrhosis. It can also happen if the bile duct becomes blocked by cancer, which causes bile produced by the liver to flow back into the bloodstream.

Jaundice makes the skin and the whites of the eyes go yellow and may make the skin very itchy. Other signs of jaundice are dark-coloured urine and pale stools (bowel motions).

Sometimes, excess fluid can build up in the abdomen and legs, which causes swelling known as ascites (Figure 36.3). Other possible symptoms include: loss of appetite, unexpected weight loss, nausea and vomiting, and pyrexia.

Management

Advise patients with liver cancer to avoid alcohol or other substances that may damage the liver. Both the patient and the family need extensive nursing support. Controlling pain is a priority.

Not all liver cancer is treatable. Time should be spent with the patient so that there is opportunity for the patient and family to express fears, thoughts and anger. As the prognosis of liver cancer is poor, the patient may have little time to put their affairs in order and to prepare for impending death. In the early stages the patient may be able to do all their activities of daily living, but as the disease progresses, they will need assistance in maintaining this.

The patient and family may benefit from referral to a cancer specialist team for support and management of pain.

Surgery

Surgery is the main treatment for primary liver cancer. Unfortunately, for many people it is not possible to remove the cancer with an operation. Sometimes a lobe of the liver may be removed. This is called a lobectomy or hemi-hepatectomy. Providing there are no other diseases, for example liver cirrhosis, the liver will regenerate.

Liver transplant is another option. If the tumours in the liver are too big, a liver transplant will not be an option. A liver transplant is not an option when the cancer has spread out of the liver. Cancer cells elsewhere in the body would be left behind even if the liver was removed. So the surgery would not cure the cancer.

Chemotherapy

Chemoembolization, also called transarterial chemoembolization (TACE), means having chemotherapy directly to the area of the liver that contains the cancer and then blocking off the blood supply to the tumour. This may be offered with surgery and radiofrequency.

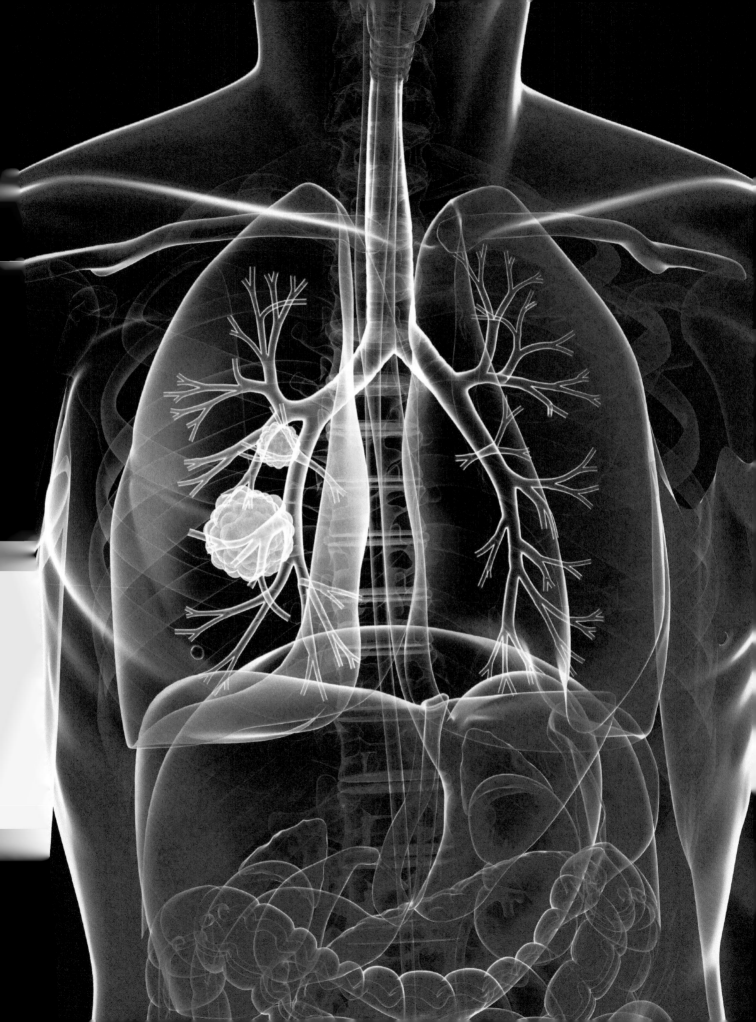

The urinary system

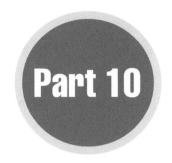

Part 10

Chapters

37 Renal failure

Figure 37.1 Renal system

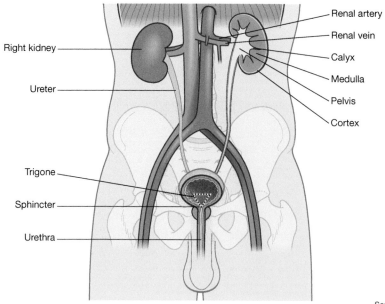

Right kidney

Ureter

Renal artery

Renal vein

Calyx

Medulla

Pelvis

Cortex

Trigone

Sphincter

Urethra

Source:
Peate, Wild & Nair, *Nursing Practice:
Knowledge and Care*, 2014

Figure 37.2 The structures of a nephron

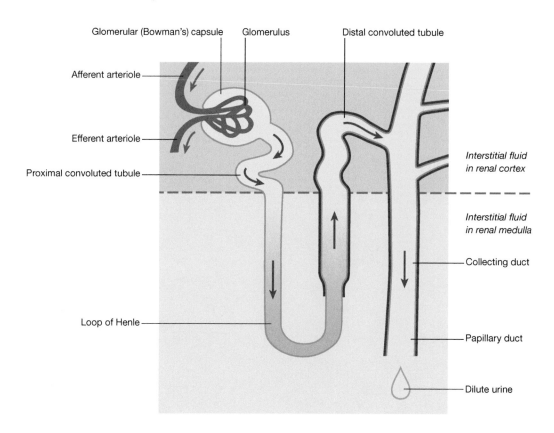

Glomerular (Bowman's) capsule

Glomerulus

Distal convoluted tubule

Afferent arteriole

Efferent arteriole

Proximal convoluted tubule

*Interstitial fluid
in renal cortex*

*Interstitial fluid
in renal medulla*

Collecting duct

Papillary duct

Loop of Henle

Dilute urine

Source: Peate I & Nair M *Fundamentals of Anatomy and Physiology for Student Nurses (2011)*

Pathophysiology for Nurses at a Glance, First Edition. Muralitharan Nair and Ian Peate. © 2015 John Wiley & Sons, Ltd. Published 2015 by John Wiley & Sons, Ltd.
Companion website: www.ataglanceseries.com/nursing/pathophysiology

Overview of anatomy and physiology

There are two kidneys, which are located in the abdominal cavity and lie at a slightly oblique angle on either side of the vertebral column at the levels of T_{12} through L_3. They are approximately 10–12 cm long, 5–7 cm wide and 3–4 cm thick. They are bean-shaped organs, where the outer surface of the kidney is convex and the inner surface is concave in shape. Near the centre of the concave border is an indentation called renal hilum through which the ureter, renal artery, renal vein, lymphatic vessels and nerves enter and exit the kidney (Figure 37.1).

The nephron is the structural and functional unit of the kidney. Each nephron functions as an independent unit and produces a miniscule quantity of urine. The nephron can be differentiated into the following regions: Bowman's capsule, glomerulus, proximal convoluted tubule, loop of Henle, distal convoluted tubule and collecting ducts (Figure 37.2).

Blood supply

The kidneys receive their blood supply directly from the aorta via the renal arteries and blood is returned to the inferior vena cava via the renal veins. The kidneys receive approximately 20% of the cardiac output. The blood supply to the kidneys arises from the paired renal arteries at the level of L_2. They enter into the renal hilum, the passageway into the kidney, with the renal vein anteriorly; the renal artery and the renal pelvis posteriorly. The renal veins return the blood from the kidneys to the renal artery at the hilum. The left renal vein is longer than the right as it crosses the midline to reach the inferior vena cava (IVC).

Functions

The kidneys serve important functions, including filtration and excretion of metabolic waste products (urea and ammonium); regulation of necessary electrolytes, fluid and acid-base balance; and stimulation of red blood cell production. They also serve to regulate blood pressure via the renin-angiotensin-aldosterone system, controlling reabsorption of water and maintaining intravascular volume. The kidneys also reabsorb glucose and amino acids and have hormonal functions via erythropoietin, calcitriol and vitamin D activation.

Pathophysiology
Acute kidney injury

AKI is a rapid deterioration of renal function, resulting in inability to maintain fluid, electrolyte and acid-base balance. It is detected and monitored by serial serum creatinine readings primarily, which rise acutely, and urine output and GFR will decrease.

Aetiology

Prerenal These include: volume depletion (e.g. haemorrhage, severe vomiting or diarrhoea, burns, inappropriate diuresis); cardiac failure;cirrhosis; nephrotic syndrome; hypotension. Renal hypoperfusion: these include non-steroidal anti-inflammatory drugs (NSAIDs) or selective cyclo-oxygenase-2 (COX-2) inhibitors; angiotensin-converting enzyme (ACE) inhibitors or angiotensin-II receptor antagonists (AIIRAs – commonly called angiotensin receptor blockers (ARBs)); abdominal aortic aneurysm; renal artery stenosis or occlusion; hepatorenal syndrome.

Intrarenal Glomerular disease: this includes glomerulonephritis; thrombosis; haemolytic uraemic syndrome. Tubular injury: this includes acute tubular necrosis (ATN) following prolonged ischaemia; nephrotoxins (e.g. aminoglycosides, radiocontrast media, myoglobin). Vascular disease: this includes vasculitis (usually associated with antineutrophil cytoplasmic antibody); cryoglobulinaemia; polyarteritis nodosa; thrombotic micro-angiopathy; cholesterol emboli; renal artery stenosis; renal vein thrombosis; malignant hypertension; eclampsia.

Postrenal This includes calculus; prostatic hypertrophy or malignancy; retroperitoneal fibrosis; bladder tumours; pelvic malignancy; urethral strictures; papillary necrosis.

Chronic kidney disease

Any condition that destroys the renal function can lead to CKD. The pathophysiology of CKD involves a gradual loss of entire nephron units. Chronic kidney disease is divided into five stages of increasing severity. In the early stages, as nephrons are slowly destroyed, remaining healthy nephrons take over the functions but become hypertrophied. The blood pressure and the filteration in the remaining healthy nephrons increase to compensate for the loss of nephrons, resulting in damage of the remaining healthy nephrons. This process of persistent loss of nephron function may continue even after the initial disease process has resolved.

Signs and symptoms

Symptoms can vary from person to person. Someone in early stage kidney disease may not feel sick or notice symptoms as they occur. When kidneys fail to filter properly, waste accumulates in the blood and the body, a condition called azotaemia. Very low levels of azotaemia may produce few, if any, symptoms. Renal failure accompanied by noticeable symptoms is termed uraemia.

Other symptoms include: weight loss; blood in the urine; vomiting and diarrhoea; swelling of the legs, ankles, feet, face and/or hands; shortness of breath due to extra fluid on the lungs; difficulty in micturition.

Management

The management of renal failure depends which type it is. A full nursing assessment of vital signs, weight, fluid intake and output, nursing history and assessment of the patient's knowledge of the disease process should all be carried out in order to provide high-quality care.

The primary focus in drug management for AKI is to restore and maintain renal perfusion and to eliminate drugs that are nephrotoxic from the treatment regimen. Adequate hydration is of paramount importance to the patient's management. Strict nutritional status should be maintained. Protein intake should be limited to minimize the increase of nitrogenous wastes. Carbohydrates are increased to maintain adequate calorie intake and provide a protein-sparing effect. Where necessary, the dietician may be involved in the care of the patient with AKI.

In CKD, unlike carbohydrates and fats, the body is unable to store excess proteins. Any unused protein is broken down as urea and nitrogenous waste, which are normally excreted by the kidneys. In CKD, these waste products are retained by the body, resulting in the toxic build-up of these waste products producing uraemic symptoms. However, prolonged dietary protein restriction should be avoided. Once the dialysis has commenced, a high protein diet is recommended. Water and sodium intake are regulated to maintain the extracellular fluid volume at normal levels. Strict water and sodium restrictions may be necessary as the CKD progresses.

38 Pyelonephritis

Figure 38.1 Anatomy of the kidney

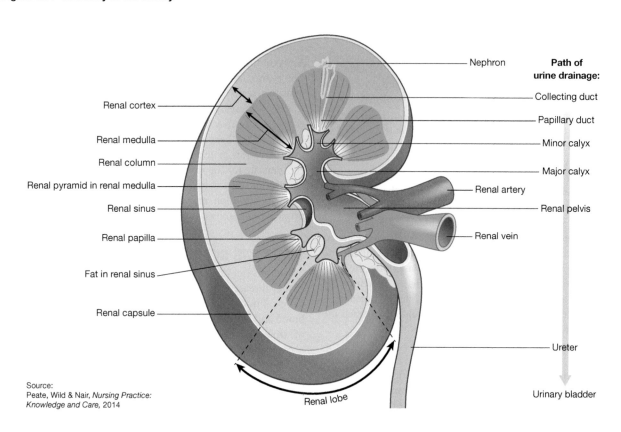

Renal cortex

Renal medulla

Renal column

Renal pyramid in renal medulla

Renal sinus

Renal papilla

Fat in renal sinus

Renal capsule

Nephron

Path of urine drainage:

Collecting duct

Papillary duct

Minor calyx

Major calyx

Renal artery

Renal pelvis

Renal vein

Renal lobe

Ureter

Urinary bladder

Source:
Peate, Wild & Nair, *Nursing Practice: Knowledge and Care*, 2014

Figure 38.2 A kidney affected by chronic pyelonephritis

Normal

Chronic pyelonephritis

Blunted calyx

Scar

Figure 38.3 Causes of hydronephrosis

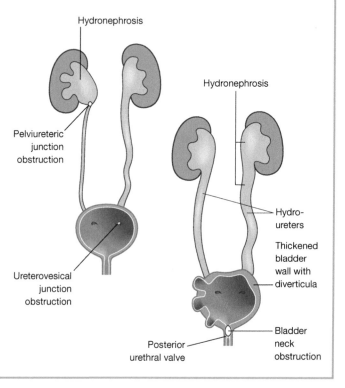

Hydronephrosis

Pelviureteric junction obstruction

Ureterovesical junction obstruction

Posterior urethral valve

Hydronephrosis

Hydro-ureters

Thickened bladder wall with diverticula

Bladder neck obstruction

Pathophysiology for Nurses at a Glance, First Edition. Muralitharan Nair and Ian Peate. © 2015 John Wiley & Sons, Ltd. Published 2015 by John Wiley & Sons, Ltd.
Companion website: www.ataglanceseries.com/nursing/pathophysiology

Overview of anatomy and physiology

There are two kidneys, one on each side of the abdomen. They make urine, which drains down the ureters into the bladder. Urine is stored in the bladder. It is passed out through the tube from the bladder (the urethra) from time to time.

What causes kidney infection?

Most kidney infections develop as a complication of a bladder infection (cystitis). Germs (bacteria) causing cystitis can sometimes travel up to infect a kidney. The bacteria are usually those which live in the bowel. They can travel from the back passage (anus) up the tube which passes out urine from the bladder (the urethra), into the bladder and cause a bladder infection. This infection can then travel up the ureter to cause a kidney infection.

Pathophysiology

Pyelonephritis relates to inflammation of the parenchyma and the pelvis of the kidney and it is usually associated with bacterial infection. Pyelonephritis can either be acute or chronic. Acute pyelonephritis is a bacterial infection of the kidney which may start from the lower urinary tract and ascend right to the kidney; chronic pyelonephritis is associated with non-bacterial infections and inflammatory processes that may be metabolic, chemical or immunological in origin.

Acute pyelonephritis

Acute pyelonephritis usually results from an infection that ascends to the kidney from the lower urinary tract. Asymptomatic bacteriuria or cystitis can lead to acute pyelonephritis. Risk factors include pregnancy (because of slowed ureteral peristalsis), urinary tract obstruction and congenital malformation. Urinary tract trauma, scarring, calculi (stones), kidney disorders such as polycystic or hypertensive kidney disease, and chronic diseases such as diabetes may also contribute to pyelonephritis. Vesico-ureteral reflux (VUR) a condition in which urine moves from the bladder back toward the kidney, is a common risk factor in children who develop pyelonephritis, and is also seen in adults when bladder outflow is obstructed.

The infection spreads from the renal pelvis to the renal cortex. The pelvis, calyces and medulla of the kidney are primarily affected, with white blood cell (WBC) infiltration and inflammation. The kidney becomes grossly oedematous. Localized abscesses may develop on the cortical surface of the kidney. As with cystitis, *E. coli* is the organism responsible for 85% of the cases of acute pyelonephritis. Other organisms commonly found include *Proteus* and *Klebsiella* bacteria that normally inhabit the intestinal tract.

Chronic pyelonephritis

Chronic pyelonephritis involves chronic inflammation and scarring of the tubules and interstitial tissues of the kidney (Figure 38.2). It is a common cause of chronic renal failure. It may develop as a result of UTIs or other conditions that damage the kidneys, such as hypertension or vascular conditions, severe vesico-ureteral reflux or obstruction of the urinary tract.

The affected kidney is smaller in size (contracted) and the surface shows coarse scarring. If both kidneys are affected appearance is asymmetrical. Biopsy of the kidney show calyces are deformed and blunted. Coarse scarring involving the cortico-medullary regions, and showing more prominently in upper and lower poles (if reflux associated) are seen. In obstruction associated cases there could be features of hydronephrosis, too (Figure 38.3).

Investigations and diagnosis

Some investigations for UTI may include: history of any previous UTI, urine culture – for high-risk patients, for example pregnant or immunosuppressed patients, or if a patient failed to respond to earlier antibiotic treatment. Urine culture should always be done in men with a history suggestive of UTI regardless of the results of the urinalysis. An ultrasound of the upper urinary tract should be carried out to rule out urinary obstruction or renal stone disease in acute uncomplicated pyelonephritis in premenopausal, non-pregnant women.

Signs and symptoms

Some of the signs and symptoms include: dysuria, urgency, nocturia, haematuria, pyrexia, tachycardia, shaking, chills (especially in pyelonephritis), flank pain (especially in pyelonephritis) and malaise (especially in pyelonephritis). While patients with chronic pyelonephritis may have acute infections, sometimes there are no symptoms, or the symptoms may be so mild that they go unnoticed. This carries the risk that the infectious inflammatory disease may progress slowly, undetected over many years until there is enough deterioration to produce kidney failure.

Urinalysis: the urine is often cloudy with an offensive smell. It may be positive on dipstick urinalysis for blood, protein, leukocyte esterase and nitrite. A midstream specimen of urine (MSU) should be sent off for microscopy and culture, although there is often poor correlation between symptoms and bacteriuria. A catheter specimen will be acceptable if a catheter is *in situ*. Microscopy of urine shows pyuria.

Blood cultures: if pyelonephritis has spread to the blood, blood cultures can detect this and guide treatment. These are positive in approximately 12–20% of patients with pyelonephritis.

Management

The main objective in UTI is to identify the cause and offer the appropriate treatment. The patient will need reassurance and psychological support and health education. The patient with acute pyelonephritis should be encouraged to be on bed rest until symptoms of pyrexia and severe groin pain subside. It is important for nurses to report signs of groin pain such as restlessness, sweating and tachycardia, for prompt action.

Antibiotics are generally prescribed for a total of at least seven days. Part of this course of treatment may be given in the hospital intravenously; the remainder of the treatment may be taken at home in the form of pills. Blood pressure should be controlled to slow the progression of renal failure. Ideally, angiotensin-converting enzyme (ACE) inhibitors should be used.

In rare cases, pyelonephritis may progress to form a pocket of infection (abscess). Abscesses are difficult or impossible to cure with antibiotics alone and must be drained. Most often, this is done with a tube inserted through the skin on the back into the kidney abscess (a procedure called a nephrostomy).

39 Renal calculi

Figure 39.1 Calcium oxalate stones

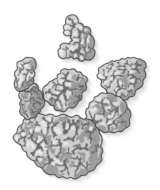

Figure 39.2 Struvite stone

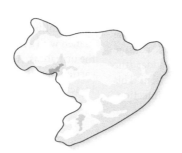

Figure 39.3 Uric acid stones

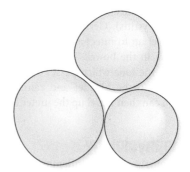

Figure 39.4 Cystine stone in the bladder

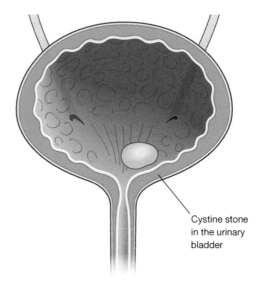

Cystine stone
in the urinary
bladder

Figure 39.5 Ultrasonic shock wave to break kidney stones

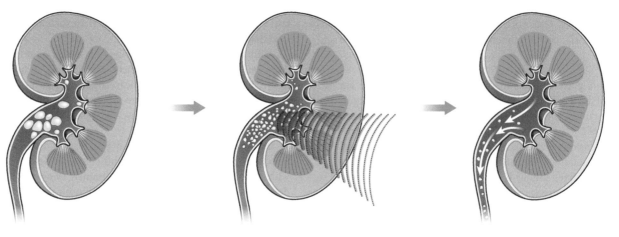

Kidney stones too large to pass
through the ureter

Ultrasound shock waves break up stones

Smaller stones pass out in urine

Pathophysiology for Nurses at a Glance, First Edition. Muralitharan Nair and Ian Peate. © 2015 John Wiley & Sons, Ltd. Published 2015 by John Wiley & Sons, Ltd.
Companion website: www.ataglanceseries.com/nursing/pathophysiology

Overview of anatomy and physiology

Normally, a balance exists in the kidneys between the need to conserve water and to eliminate poorly soluble materials such as calcium salts. This balance is affected by factors such as diet, environmental temperature and activity. Protective inorganic and organic substances in the urine, such as pyrophosphate, citrate and glycoproteins, normally inhibit stone formation.

Renal calculi are formed when the urine is supersaturated with salt and minerals such as calcium oxalate, struvite (ammonium magnesium phosphate), uric acid and cystine. Approximately 60–80% of stones contain calcium. They vary considerably in size from small 'gravel-like' stones, to large staghorn calculi. The calculi may stay in the position in which they are formed, or migrate down the urinary tract, producing symptoms along the way.

Although the majority of stones are idiopathic, a number of risk factors have been identified. The greatest risk factor for stone formation is a prior personal or family history of urinary calculi. A genetic predisposition towards the accumulation of certain mineral substances in the urine or a congenital lack of protective factors may explain the familial link. Other identified risk factors include dehydration, with resultant increased urine concentration, immobility and excess dietary intake of calcium, oxalate or proteins. Gout, hyperparathyroidism and urinary stasis or repeated infections also contribute to calculus formation.

Pathophysiology

Three factors contribute to urolithiasis: supersaturation, nucleation and lack of inhibitory substances in the urine. When the concentration of an insoluble salt in the urine is very high, that is, when the urine is supersaturated, crystals may form. Usually, these crystals disperse and are eliminated because the bonds holding them together are weak. However, a nucleus of crystals may develop stable bonds to form a stone. More often, crystals form around an organic matrix or mucoprotein nucleus to become a stone. The stimulus required to initiate crystallization in supersaturated urine may be minimal. Ingesting a meal high in insoluble salt, or decreased fluid intake as occurs during sleep, allows the concentration to increase to the point where precipitation occurs and stones are formed and grow. When fluid intake is adequate, no stone growth occurs. The acidity or alkalinity of the urine and the presence or absence of calculus-inhibiting compounds, affect lithiasis.

Most (75–80%) kidney stones are calcium stones, composed of calcium oxalate and/or calcium phosphate. These stones are generally associated with high concentrations of calcium in the blood or urine. Uric acid stones develop when the urine concentration of uric acid is high. They are more common in men, and may be associated with gout. Genetic factors contribute to the development of uric acid stones and calcium stones. Struvite stones are associated with UTI caused by urease-producing bacteria such as *Proteus*. These stones can grow to become very large, filling the renal pelvis and calyces. They often are called staghorn stones because of their shape. Cystine stones are rare, and are associated with a genetic defect.

Calcium stones: most kidney stones are calcium stones, usually in the form of calcium oxalate (Figure 39.1). Oxalate is a naturally occurring substance found in food. Some fruits and vegetables, as well as nuts and chocolate, have high oxalate levels. The liver also produces oxalate. Dietary factors, high doses of vitamin D, intestinal bypass surgery and several metabolic disorders can increase the concentration of calcium or oxalate in urine. Calcium stones may also occur in the form of calcium phosphate.

Struvite stones: struvite stones form in response to an infection, such as a urinary tract infection (Figure 39.2). These stones can grow quickly and become quite large, sometimes with few symptoms or little warning.

Uric acid stones: uric acid stones can form in people who don't drink enough fluids or who lose too much fluid, those who eat a high-protein diet, and those who have gout (Figure 39.3). Certain genetic factors also may increase the risk of uric acid stones.

Cystine stones: these stones form in people with a hereditary disorder that causes the kidneys to excrete too much of certain amino acids (cystinuria) (Figure 39.4).

Signs and symptoms

A kidney stone may not cause symptoms until it moves around within the kidney or passes into the ureter – the tube connecting the kidney and bladder. At that point, these signs and symptoms may occur: pain on urination, cloudy and foul smelling urine, haematuria, fever and chills if an infection is present, nausea and vomiting, and a persistent urge to urinate. Pain caused by a kidney stone may change – for instance shifting to a different location or increasing in intensity – as the stone moves through the urinary tract.

Management

Treatment for kidney stones varies, depending on the type of stone and the cause. Most kidney stones won't require invasive treatment.

Drinking water: encourage the patient to drink 2–2.5 litres a day to help flush out the urinary system. Unless otherwise informed, drink enough fluid – mostly water – to produce clear or nearly clear urine.

Analgesia: passing a small stone can cause some discomfort. To relieve mild pain, the doctor may recommend pain relievers such as ibuprofen.

Antibiotics: in some cases, if the urine is infected the doctor may prescribe suitable antibiotics to treat the infection.

Kidney stones that can't be treated with conservative measures – either because they're too large to pass on their own or because they cause bleeding, kidney damage or ongoing urinary tract infections – may require more invasive treatment. For example, extracorporeal shock wave lithotripsy (ESWL), laser lithotripsy and percutaneous ultrasonic lithotripsy (Figure 39.5).

40 Bladder cancer

Figure 40.1 Urinary bladder

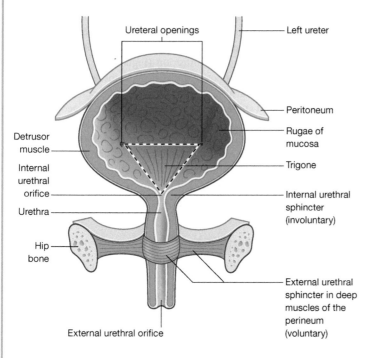

Source:
Peate, Wild & Nair, *Nursing Practice:
Knowledge and Care,* 2014

Figure 40.2 Male urethra

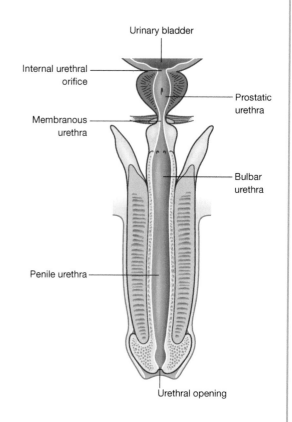

Figure 40.3 Female urethra

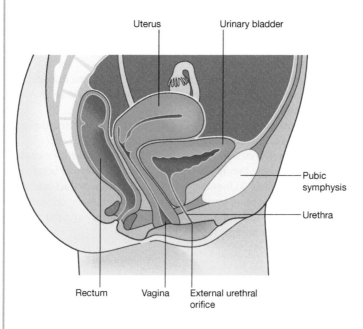

Source:
Peate, Wild & Nair, *Nursing Practice:
Knowledge and Care,* 2014

Figure 40.4 Staging of bladder cancer

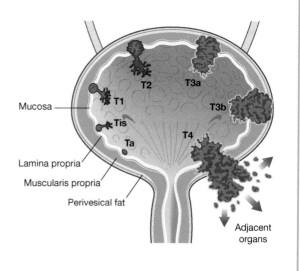

Source:
Peate, Wild & Nair, *Nursing Practice:
Knowledge and Care,* 2014

Overview of anatomy and physiology

The urinary bladder is a muscular sac in the pelvis, just above and behind the pubic bone. When empty, the bladder is about the size and shape of a pear.

Urine is made in the kidneys, and travels down two tubes called ureters to the bladder. The bladder stores urine, allowing urination to be infrequent and voluntary. The bladder is lined by layers of muscle tissue that stretch to accommodate urine. The normal capacity of the bladder is 400–600 mL.

In the floor of the bladder is a small triangular area called the trigone. The trigone is formed by the two ureteral orifices and the internal urethral orifice. The area is very sensitive to expansion and once stretched to a certain degree, the urinary bladder signals the brain of its need to empty. The signals become stronger as the bladder continues to fill. During urination, the bladder muscles contract, and two sphincters (valves) open to allow urine to flow out. Urine exits the bladder into the urethra, which carries urine out of the body.

The flow of urine through the urethra is controlled by the internal and external urethral sphincter muscles. The internal urethral sphincter is made of smooth muscle and opens involuntarily when the bladder reaches a certain set level of distention. The opening of the internal sphincter results in the sensation of needing to urinate. The external urethral sphincter is made of skeletal muscle and may be opened to allow urine to pass through the urethra or may be held closed to delay urination.

Urethra

The male urethra is a narrow fibromuscular tube that conducts urine and semen from the bladder and ejaculatory ducts, respectively, to the exterior of the body (see the image). Although the male urethra is a single structure, it is composed of a heterogeneous series of segments: prostatic, membranous and spongy. Because it passes through the penis, the urethra is longer in men (approximately 20 cm) (Figure 40.2) than in women (approximately 3–5 cm) (Figure 40.3).

Pathophysiology

Cancer is a disease of the cells in the body. The body is made up from millions of tiny cells. There are many different types of cell in the body, and there are many different types of cancer which arise from different types of cell. What all types of cancer have in common is that the cancer cells are abnormal and multiply out of control. A malignant tumour is a lump of tissue made from cancer cells which continue to multiply. Malignant tumours can invade into nearby tissues and organs, which can cause damage.

Malignant tumours may also spread to other parts of the body. This happens if some cells break off from the first (primary) tumour and are carried in the bloodstream or lymph channels to other parts of the body. These small groups of cells may then multiply to form secondary tumours (metastases) in one or more parts of the body. These secondary tumours may then grow, invade and damage nearby tissues, and spread again.

Some cancers are more serious than others; some are more easily treated than others (particularly if diagnosed at an early stage); some have a better outlook (prognosis) than others. See Figure 40.4 for staging of bladder tumours.

Signs and symptoms

Blood in the urine: this is the most common symptom of bladder cancer and occurs in the vast majority of people with bladder cancer. Having blood in the urine does not necessarily mean a person has cancer, since other conditions (including infections) can lead to bloody urine, but blood in the urine is never normal and should always be evaluated by a doctor. Other symptoms include loss of appetite and weight, back or abdominal pain and pain on micturition.

Management

Treatment depends on the position and size of the cancer in the bladder and how far it has spread.

Non-surgical

Transurethral resection of bladder tumour (TURBT)

TURBT is the main treatment option for early stage bladder cancer that hasn't spread into the bladder wall. TURBT is usually followed by bladder treatment with mitomycin C or Bacille Calmette-Guérin (BCG) to destroy any remaining cancer cells and reduce the chance of cancer coming back.

Bladder treatment with mitomycin C or Bacille Calmette-Guérin (BCG)

Mitomycin C is a chemotherapy medicine used to destroy cancer cells. BCG is an immunotherapy that contains a weak form of the bacterium *Mycobacterium bovis* that works by encouraging the immune system to attack cancer cells.

Surgical

Removing the bladder and surrounding tissues is the main treatment for muscle-invasive bladder cancer. The operation is called a complete or radical cystectomy. If a tumour has grown into the wall of the bladder but has not spread to other organs, treatment usually involves surgical removal of the tumour, or combined chemotherapy and radiation therapy.

Chemotherapy and radiation therapy

Radiation is another adjunctive therapy used in the treatment of urinary tumours. Although radiation alone is not curative, it can reduce tumour size prior to surgery and is used as palliative treatment for inoperable tumours and persons who cannot tolerate surgery. Radiation therapy also is used in combination with systemic chemotherapy to improve local and distant relapse rates. If radiation or chemotherapy is planned as adjunctive therapy, the patient may experience hair loss, stomatitis, nausea and vomiting, or other disturbing side effects of therapy. Nurses should be sensitive to the patient's feelings, actively listening and responding to their concerns.

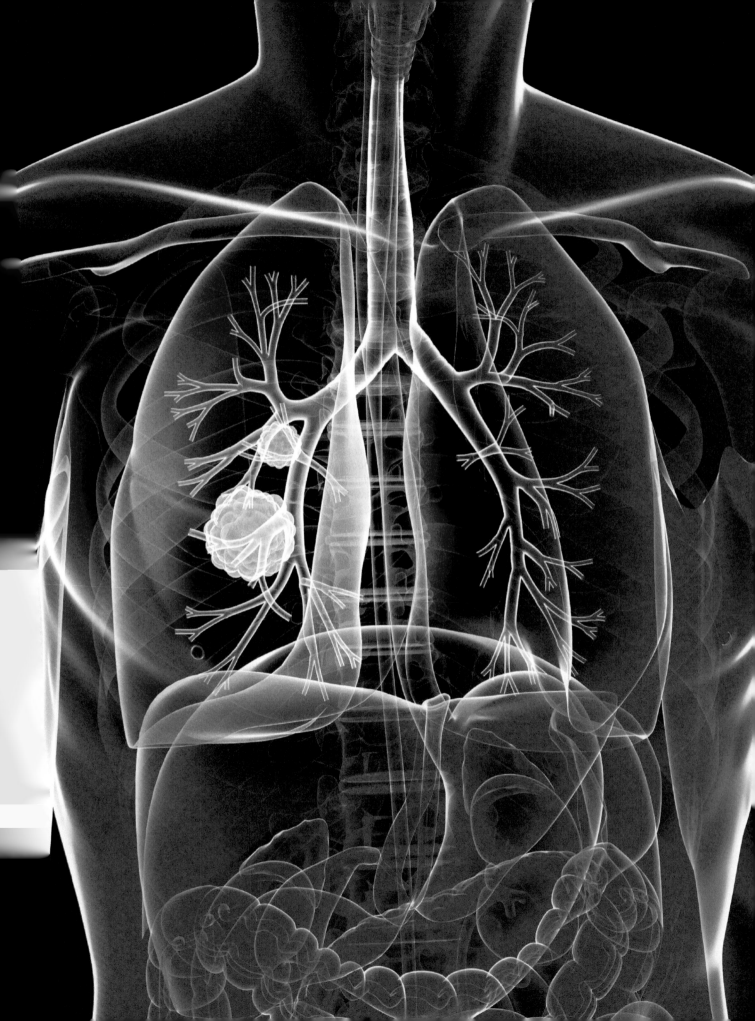

Prostate cancer

Most prostate cancers are adenocarcinomas arising in the peripheral zone of the prostate gland (see Figure 44.2). The majority of prostate cancers are slow growing, but some prostate cancers are aggressive. When prostate cancer occurs in younger men it is often more aggressive. In the UK, cancer of the prostate is currently the second most common cause of cancer death in men (lung cancer is the most common).

Pathophysiology

The aetiology of prostate cancer is unknown, genetic and environmental factors are thought to play a role; the cancer is not thought to be related to benign prostatic hyperplasia. BRCA 1 and BRCA 2 genes are important risk factors for breast and ovarian cancers, and have been implicated in prostate cancer risk. They are linked to the aggressive form of prostate cancer; knowing this will have implications for treatment.

The risk of prostate cancer increases with age. Risk factors can be seen in Figure 44.1. Male hormones affect the growth of the prostate and prostate cancer seems to be related to life-long levels of testosterone; they are testosterone dependent until late in the course of the disease.

Prostate cancer can be spread by local extension by the lymphatics or via the bloodstream. The most common sites for metastases are bone and lymph nodes.

Signs and symptoms
Symptoms

The symptoms of growths in the prostate are similar, be they benign or malignant. Early stage prostate cancers can be asymptomatic. Lower urinary symptoms, for example urinary frequency, hesitancy, nocturia and slow stream do not increase the risk of prostate cancer.

Local disease
Raised prostate specific antigen; weak stream; hesitancy; sensation of incomplete emptying; urinary frequency; urgency; urge incontinence; urinary tract infection.

Locally invasive disease
Haematuria; dysuria; incontinence; haematospermia; perineal and suprapubic pain; obstruction of ureters; loin pain; anuria; symptoms of renal failure; erectile dysfunction; rectal symptoms such as tenesmus

Metastatic disease
Bone pain or sciatica; paraplegia secondary to spinal cord compression; lymphadenopathy; loin pain or anuria due to ureteric obstruction by lymph nodes; lethargy (anaemia, uraemia); weight loss; cachexia.

Advanced disease: malaise; bone pain; anorexia; weight loss; obstructive nephropathy; paralysis due to cord compression; abdominal palpation may demonstrate a palpable bladder due to outflow obstruction.

Signs

Digital rectal examination (DRE) may reveal a hard, irregular gland. Indications of possible prostate cancer are: asymmetry of the gland, nodule within one lobe, induration of part or all of the prostate. lack of mobility – adhesion to surrounding tissue, palpable seminal vesicles.

Physical examination only cannot reliably differentiate benign prostatic disease from cancer. A biopsy is needed to establish a diagnosis; multiple biopsies may be needed before prostate cancer is detected. If cancer is suspected, determining whether the disease is localized or extends outside the capsule is essential for planning treatment. Locally advanced disease is often indicated by obliteration of the lateral sulcus or involvement of the seminal vesical. Findings in men with advanced disease can include: cancer cachexia, bony tenderness, lower-extremity lymphoedema or deep venous thrombosis, adenopathy, overdistended bladder. Neurological examination, including determination of external anal sphincter tone, helps detect possible spinal cord compression. See Figure 44.3 for digital rectal examination findings.

Investigations

Screening for prostate cancer is a contentious topic. DRE and PSA evaluation are the two components used in prostate cancer screening. Transrectal ultrasonography (TRUS) has been linked with a high false-positive rate, which makes it unsuitable as a screening tool. However, it has an established role in directing prostatic biopsies. See Figure 44.3 for investigations used in prostate cancer.
- PSA assessment (see Figure 44.4)
- Digital rectal examination
- Rectal ultrasound
- Needle biopsy
- Template biopsy
- Intravenous urogram
    Other tests:
- Bone scan
- X-rays
- MRI CT scans
- Abdominal ultra sound

Management

Staging of the cancer determines how far the cancer has spread. The various investigations provide information about the stage and this helps decide on treatment options.

Low-risk localized prostate cancer

If the tumour is small and well differentiated, active monitoring or active surveillance monitors the cancer to see whether it begins to develop.

High-risk localized prostate cancer

This refers to cancer that has broken through to the prostatic capsule.

A number of approaches can be offered to the man but these depend on the stage of the disease (the TNM staging system is used), this includes the presence (or not) of metastatic spread as well as the man's own choice. It is essential all options are offered to the man and an informed decision is reached. Treatment options may be used in isolation or a combined approach may be used. Options will include:
- Surgery: radical prostatectomy (robot assisted, retropubic, perineal, laparoscopic)
- Radiotherapy: external beam radiation therapy
- Brachytherapy
- Hormone therapy (androgen depravation therapy)
- Cryotherapy
- High frequency ultrasound therapy
- Orchidectomy (androgen depravation therapy)
- Chemotherapy
- Palliative care

45 Testicular cancer

Figure 45.1 Royal Marsden staging of testicular tumours

- **I – No evidence of disease outside the testis**

- **IM – As above but with persistently raised tumour markers**

- **II – Infradiaphragmatic nodal involvement:**
  IIA – maximum diameter <2 cm
  IIB – maximum diameter 2–5 cm
  IIC – maximum diameter >5–10 cm
  IID – maximum diameter >10 cm

- **III – Supradiaphragmatic and infradiaphragmatic node involvement:**
  – abdominal nodes A, B, C, as above
  – mediastinal nodes M+
  – neck nodes N+

- **IV – Extralymphatic metastases:**
  – abdominal nodes A, B, C, as above
  – mediastinal or neck nodes as for stage III
  – lungs:
    - L1 <3 metastases
    - L2 multiple metastases <2 cm maximum diameter
    - L3 multiple metastases >2 cm in diameter
  – Liver involvement H+

Figure 45.2 Pelvic and para-aortic lymph nodes

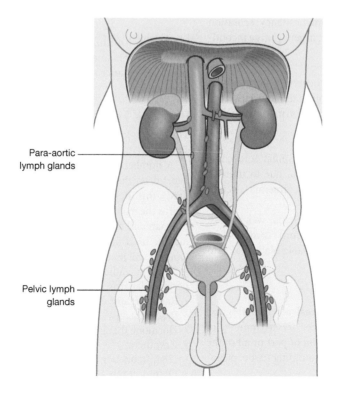

Para-aortic lymph glands

Pelvic lymph glands

Source:
Peate, Wild & Nair, *Nursing Practice: Knowledge and Care*, 2014

In the UK, primary testicular tumours are the most common solid malignant tumour in men aged between 20 and 35 years. Testicular cancer is rare. With timely diagnosis, testicular cancer is highly treatable and usually curable. Testicular cancers are sensitive to chemotherapy and even when metastatic are curable, it is the most treatable form of urological cancer.

Testicular cancer

Approximately 50% of all cases occur in men under 35; testicular cancer rarely occurs before puberty. It is the most common cancer in men aged 15–44 years. The incidence of this cancer has increased over the years and the reasons for this are unknown.

Pathophysiology

The cause of testicular cancer is unknown. The majority of testicular tumours arise from the germ cells. Testicular germ cell tumours can be subdivided into seminoma and non-seminomatous germ cell tumours. Half of all germ cell tumours are non-seminomas and about 45% seminomas. The non-germ cell tumours include Leydig cell tumours, Sertoli cell tumours and sarcomas.

There are a number of risk factors associated with testicular cancer: cryptorchidism, Klinefelter's syndrome, family history, infertility, low birth weight, young maternal and paternal age, multi-parity, breach delivery, infantile hernia, taller men and testicular microlithiasis on ultrasound. A genetic factor is that most testicular tumours display an abnormality on chromosome 12. Possession of the testicular germ cell tumour 1 (TGCT1) gene on the man's X chromosome gene may increase risk of testicular malignancy by up to 50 times. The risk for the disease is higher in first-degree relatives of men with testicular cancer than in the general population. Siblings are at particularly increased risk, as are sons of affected men.

Testicular cancers metastasize in particular fashion, to the retroperineal lymph nodes, with subsequent involvement of the mediastinal lymph nodes, lungs and liver.

Signs and symptoms

Until proven otherwise, any lump or firm area within the testicle should be considered a potential tumour.

Localized disease

The most common presenting symptom is a painless swelling or nodule of one testicle; a lump is palpable in nearly all cases. During physical examination this mass/nodule cannot be separated from the testes. Men with atrophic testes will feel enlargement. There may be a dull ache or heavy sensation in the lower abdomen, and men may complain of a dragging sensation. Men who experience a haematoma with trauma should undergo evaluation in order to rule out testicular cancer as it is probably the trauma that leads the man to examine himself and find the tumour as opposed to being the reason of malignant change.

Metastatic disease

In disseminated disease there are symptoms of lymphatic or haematogenous spread. There may be a neck mass in supraclavicular lymph node, metastatic disease, anorexia, nausea and other gastrointestinal symptoms. Bulky retroperitoneal disease may be felt as back pain. Cough, chest pain, haemoptysis and shortness of breath could be a presenting symptom of mediastinal adenopathy or lung metastasis.

Gynaecomastia may occur in some men with testicular germ cell tumours that produce human chorionic gonadotropin (hCG), such as choriocarcinoma, and is a systemic manifestation. Marked overproduction of hCG can develop hyperthyroidism since hCG and thyroid stimulating hormone have a common alpha-subunit and a beta-subunit with considerable homology.

Men who present with a scrotal swelling should be examined carefully and attempts made to discriminate between lumps arising from the testes and other intrascrotal swellings. In order to make the distinction an ultrasound scan should be performed.

Investigations

Investigations will include an assay of tumour markers (see below), bilateral testicular ultrasound and chest X-ray.

Confirmation of diagnosis is usually by ultrasound. Histology can follow an inguinal orchidectomy (pathological diagnosis). Staging of the disease can be undertaken by thoraco-abdominal CT scanning.

Tumour markers are useful in staging and assessing response to treatment:
- Alpah-fetoprotein (AFP) is produced by yolk sac elements but not produced by seminomas.
- Beta-hCG is produced by trophoblastic elements, there may be elevated levels in teratomas and seminomas.
- Lactate dehydrogenase (LDH) should also be measured, particularly in advanced tumours.

The Royal Marsden staging of testicular tumours is used (see Figure 45.1) to stage the cancer.

Management

Management will depend on the type of tumour and its stage and is based on national guidelines. Referral to a specialist centre for the management of testicular tumours is required.

An inguinal orchidectomy should be performed where possible. All men should be offered testicular prosthesis and when appropriate arrangements should be made for sperm storage for those men who may require chemotherapy or radiotherapy.

Where there are metastases and the diagnosis is not in doubt (for example there are high tumour markers and the presence of a testicular mass) referral for immediate chemotherapy should be made.

In most cases inguinal orchidectomy is required, with removal of the testes, the tunica and spermatic cord. Retroperineal lymph node dissection can be performed after orchidectomy in non-seminomas; this is done for staging and therapeutic purposes. Surgery does have potential complications; there may be infertility and ejaculatory dysfunction.

Men with seminoma may have radiotherapy to retroperitoneal lymph glands.

Chemotherapy can help prevent non-seminoma (teratoma) returning after orchidectomy. It is used to treat any extra-testicular cancer and to treat testicular cancer returning after initial chemotherapy. When there is para-aortic lymph gland involvement chemotherapy may be recommended (see Figure 45.1.).

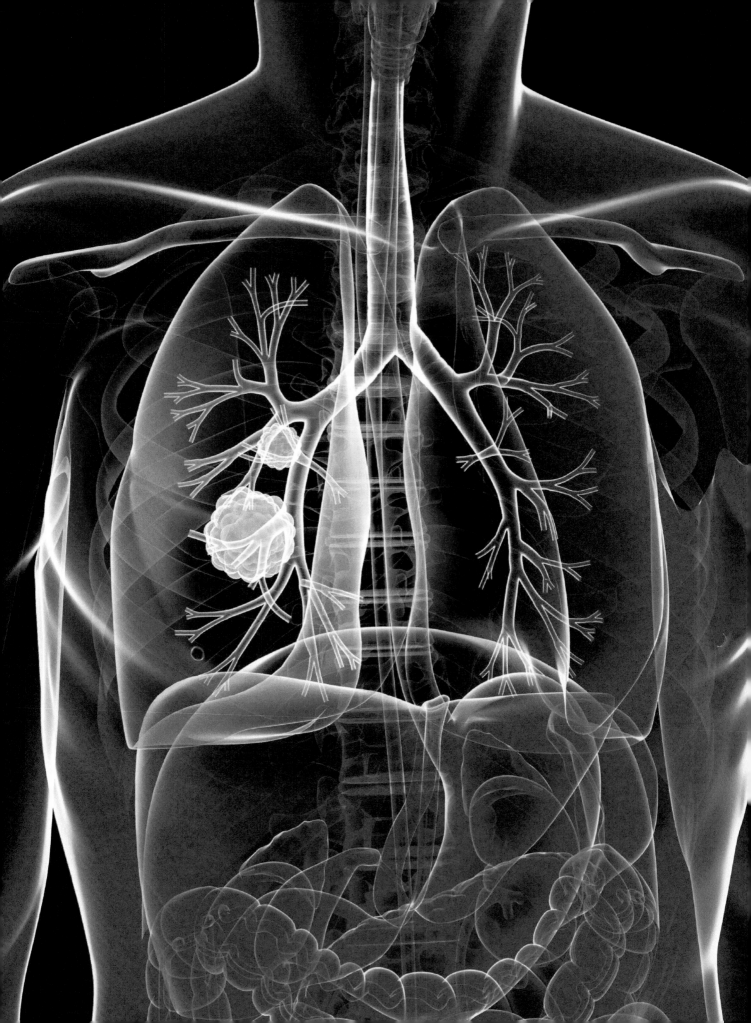

Menorrhagia refers to menstrual blood loss that interferes with a woman's physical, emotional, social and material quality of life; this can occur alone or in combination with other symptoms. The aim of any intervention should be to improve a woman's quality of life. A monthly menstrual blood loss in excess of 80 ml is said to be menorrhagia.

Menorrhagia

The average menstrual cycle has a blood loss for 7 days of a cycle of between 21 and 35 days (K = 7/21–35, where K represents menstrual cycle). For the first few days menstrual loss is heaviest, then it becomes much lighter and tails off towards the end. Other definitions include:
- Metrorrhagia – menstrual flow at irregular intervals
- Menometrorrhagia – flow that is frequent and excessive
- Polymenorrhoea – bleeding at intervals less than 21 days
- Dysfunctional uterine bleeding – abnormal uterine bleeding with no obvious structural or systemic pathology
- Dysmenorrhoea – the experience of pain with menstruation

The normal menstrual blood loss is approximately 35–40 ml. As menorrhagia is very subjective, a more practical definition may be that it is menstrual loss that is greater than the woman feels she can reasonably manage. Heavy menstrual loss is excessive blood loss that interferes with a woman's physical, social, emotional and/ or quality of life.

Pathophysiology

Approximately half of those women who complain of excessive bleeding have no pathology; this is known as dysfunctional uterine bleeding. Approximately 20% of cases are associated with anovulatory cycles and these are most common at the extremes of reproductive life. Local causes can include:
- Fibroids
- Endometrial polyps
- Adenomyosis
- Endometritis
- Endometrial hyperplasia
- Pelvic inflammatory disease
- Endometrial carcinoma

Systemic disease can include hypothyroidism, liver or kidney failure and bleeding disorders. An IUD can increase menstrual flow.

Signs and symptoms

Symptoms related by the woman with menorrhagia may often be more instructive than laboratory tests. It is essential to undertake a detailed patient history. Figure 47.1 outlines some essential issues that should be addressed in the history-taking phase.

The physical examination should be modified in order to meet the needs of the woman. The clinician should observe for signs of severe anaemia, this may confirm the patient's history of very heavy bleeding and prompt immediate in-patient care. Obesity is an independent risk factor for endometrial cancer. Adipose tissue is ideal for oestrogen conversion. Signs of androgen excess (hirsutism) may be PCOS, leading to anovulatory

bleeding. Ecchymosis is usually a sign of trauma or a bleeding disorder; purpura is also a sign of trauma or a possible bleeding disorder. Uterine size, shape and contour should be assessed. Adnexal tenderness or masses could indicate ovarian cancer; intermenstrual bleeding may be its only symptom. Finding an adnexal mass should prompt an immediate pelvic ultrasound.

Investigations

A full blood count is required (menorrhagaia is the most common cause of iron deficiency anaemia in women). Tests for endocrine irregularities, including thyroid function tests, may be needed. If there is a clinical suspicion, then undertake an assessment of bleeding disorders. Biopsy should be carried out in order to exclude endometrial cancer or atypical hyperplasia. A trans-vaginal ultrasound is the first-line diagnostic tool for identifying structural abnormalities such as fibroids. Cervical specimens should be taken if the woman is at risk of an infection.

Management

Pharmaceutical treatment is the preferred treatment; when first-line pharmacology treatment is ineffective then a second pharmaceutical treatment should be considered as opposed to an immediate referral to surgery. Medical therapy for menorrhagia should be tailored to the individual. Factors taken into consideration when selecting the appropriate medical treatment include the patient's age, coexisting medical diseases, family history and desire for fertility.

The woman must be at the centre of all decisions being made.

Pharmacology

Iron deficiency should be corrected with oral iron. The levonorgestrel intrauterine system is first-line treatment, it is a long-term treatment, left *in situ* for at least 12 months.

Consider giving tranexamic acid, mefanamic acid or the combined oral contraceptive pill if the intrauterine system is unacceptable to the woman. A 3–4 month course of a gonadotrophin-releasing hormone analogue should be considered prior to hysterectomy or myomectomy. There is no consensus about which regimens are the most effective.

Surgical options

The type of surgical intervention will depend on uterine size and the woman's desire to retain her uterus.

Endometrial ablation is the recommended first-line surgical treatment. This involves removing the full thickness of the endometrium, together with the superficial myometrium; it retains the uterus, but is contraindicated in women with large fibroids or suspected malignancy and in those who have not completed their family.

Uterine artery embolization or hysteroscopic myomectomy can be offered if the woman wishes to retain her uterus.

If the patient does not wish to retain her uterus, then vaginal hysterectomy is the first considerationa, then abdominal hysterectomy with conservation of ovaries, if appropriate.

48 Breast cancer

Figure 48.1 The female breast

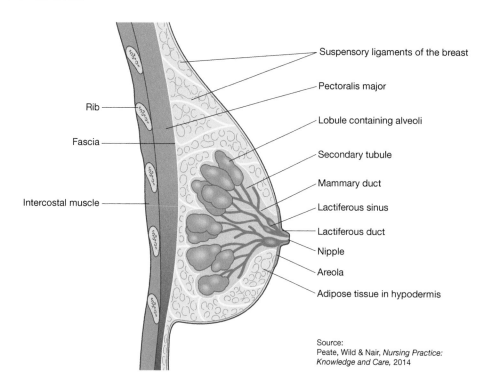

Suspensory ligaments of the breast

Pectoralis major

Lobule containing alveoli

Secondary tubule

Mammary duct

Lactiferous sinus

Lactiferous duct

Nipple

Areola

Adipose tissue in hypodermis

Rib

Fascia

Intercostal muscle

Source:
Peate, Wild & Nair, *Nursing Practice:
Knowledge and Care,* 2014

Figure 48.2 Risk factors

- Age (increases with age)
- Reproductive history
- Endogenous and exogenous hormones
- Breast density
- Previous breast disease
  – the genes BRCA1, BRCA2 and TP53 mutations
  carry very high risk. Family history, a first-degree
  relative, is the most widely recognized breast
  cancer risk factor
- Non-reproductive lifestyle

Table 48.1 Breast cancer staging

Stage 0	Carcinoma *in situ* and is not invasive
Stage I	Tumour up to 2 cm in diameter and no lymph node involvement or metastasis
Stage II	Tumour 2–5 cm in diameter or there is spread to the axillary lymph nodes on the same side and the nodes are not adherent
Stage IIIa	The tumour is over 5 cm in diameter or the nodes are adherent
Stage IIIb	Invasive breast cancer in which a tumour of any size has spread to the breast skin, chest wall or internal mammary lymph nodes and includes inflammatory breast cancer with peau d'orange
Stage IV	Is spread beyond the breast, axilla and internal mammary nodes. It may have spread to supraclavicular nodes, bone, liver, lung or brain

Pathophysiology for Nurses at a Glance, First Edition. Muralitharan Nair and Ian Peate. © 2015 John Wiley & Sons, Ltd. Published 2015 by John Wiley & Sons, Ltd.
Companion website: www.ataglanceseries.com/nursing/pathophysiology

Globally, breast cancer is the most frequently diagnosed life-threatening cancer in women and is the leading cause of cancer death among women. Breast cancer can be discovered while *in situ* (localized) or as a malignant neoplasm (spreading).

The female breasts

An adult woman's breasts are milk-producing glands on the front of the chest wall, resting on the pectoralis major, supported by and attached to the front of the chest wall on either side of the sternum by ligaments. There are 15–20 lobes arranged in a circular fashion in each breast. Each lobe comprises many lobules, with glands that produce milk in response to hormones (see Figure 48.1).

A number of early breast carcinomas are asymptomatic, particularly if they are discovered during a breast-screening programme. Larger tumours can present as a painless mass. Pain or discomfort is not usually a symptom of breast cancer.

A large number of breast cancer cases in the UK can be explained by factors that influence exposure to oestrogen, including reproductive and hormonal factors, obesity, alcohol and physical activity. Breast cancers are predominantly linked to modifiable lifestyle and environmental factors (see Figure 48.2).

Pathophysiology

The majority of breast cancers arise from either the epithelial lining of ducts, known as ductal, or from the epithelium of the terminal ducts of the lobules and these are called lobular. Carcinoma can be invasive or *in situ*. Most cancers arise from intermediate ducts and are invasive. They eventually grow through the wall of the duct and into the fatty tissue.

Current understanding of breast cancer is that invasive cancers arise through a series of molecular alterations at the cell level. These alterations result in breast epithelial cells with remarkable features and uncontrolled growth.

An infiltrating carcinoma of the nipple epithelium, called Paget's disease of the breast, accounts for approximately 1% of all breast cancers. Inflammatory carcinoma exists in less than 3% of all cases; there is a rapidly growing, sometimes painful mass increasing the breast and causing the skin covering it to become red and warm. There may be widespread infiltration of tumour.

Staging of the tumour

Tumour size, lymph node status and distant metastasis are taken into account when staging the tumour (see Table 48.1). The various tests and investigations required to make a diagnosis can also give some information about the stage. Understanding the stage is important as this helps the clinician to decide on the most appropriate treatment.

Signs and symptoms

Most early breast carcinomas are asymptomatic, especially if discovered during a breast-screening programme. Larger tumours may present as a painless mass. Pain (mastalgia) or discomfort is not usually a symptom of breast cancer; only 5% of women with a malignant mass have breast pain.

Most women will have felt a lump, there may be nipple change and in some cases nipple discharge; skin contour changes can occur. Intraduct carcinoma can present as a bloody discharge from the nipple.

Investigations

A variety of investigations are used; however, evaluation starts with an ordered inquiry that begins with symptoms and a general clinical history, along with a physical examination of the breasts, the axillary and cervical lymph nodes. Once the examination has been concluded other investigations may be required; these are used to make a diagnosis and to help with staging. Investigations should be aligned to local national guidance. Triple assessment includes the following components, clinical examination, imaging (including mammography, ultrasonography or both) and needle biopsy.

Mammography is more appropriate for less dense breasts and is almost always undertaken; ultrasound and mammography can detect more invasive tumours. Ultrasound is effective particularly when breast tissue is dense; in the younger woman it can be diagnostically more useful than mammography. MRI is used in women with dense breast tissue, cases of familial breast cancer associated with BRCA mutations, silicone gel implants, positive axillary lymph node status with occult primary tumour in the breast or if multiple tumour foci are suspected.

Core needle biopsy (image-guided) should be obtained before any surgery. Ultrasound or stereotactic mammographic guidance can be used. Open biopsy (needle localization), radio-opaque needles are used to guide biopsy (this can be done under local anaesthetic). Where there are palpable lesions fine-needle aspiration is required. Core needle biopsy is usually used for larger lesions. Excision biopsy (under local anaesthesia) allows the entire lesion to be removed). Incisional biopsy provides for part of a lesion to be removed (lesions 4 cm or larger).

Specific staging investigations include routine blood tests, such as liver function tests, chest X-ray; if metastases are suspected a CT scan is needed. Bone scintigraphy is required if there are distant metastases. Positron emission tomography can detect distant metastases.

Management

Treatment must be patient-centred, acknowledging the woman's individual needs and preferences. Discussion and involvement of the woman's family should, with their consent, be enabled. Prognosis of patients with breast cancer depends on biological characteristics of the cancer, the patient and on appropriate therapy.

The primary treatment for early stage breast cancer is surgery; many women are cured with surgery alone. The aim of breast cancer surgery includes complete resection of the primary tumour with negative margins, reducing the risk of local recurrences, and pathological staging of the tumour and axillary lymph nodes providing necessary prognostic information.

Adjuvant treatment of breast cancer is intended to treat micrometastatic disease (breast cancer cells escaping into the breast and regional lymph nodes but which have not yet had an established identifiable metastasis).

Adjuvant treatment involves radiation therapy and a number of chemotherapeutic and biological agents. Treatment attempts to reduce the risk of future recurrence, and in so doing reduce breast cancer-related morbidity and mortality.

49 Cervical cancer

Figure 49.1   Squamocolumnar junction of the cervix

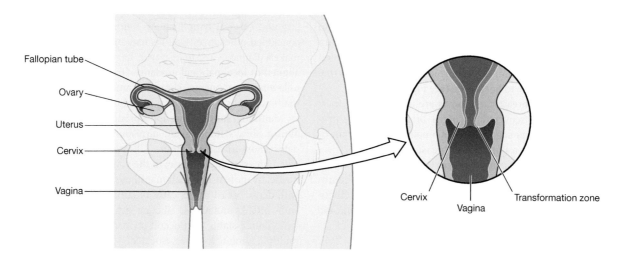

Figure 49.2   Cervical intra-epithelial neoplasia

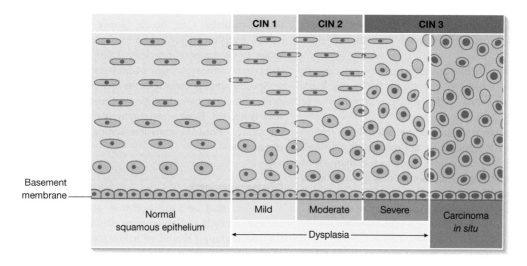

Figure 49.3   Cone biopsy

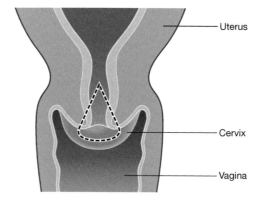

Pathophysiology for Nurses at a Glance, First Edition. Muralitharan Nair and Ian Peate. © 2015 John Wiley & Sons, Ltd. Published 2015 by John Wiley & Sons, Ltd.
Companion website: www.ataglanceseries.com/nursing/pathophysiology

Cervical cancer

Cancer of the cervix is one of the few preventable cancers; it is the most common cancer in women under 35 years old. Globally, cervical cancer is the second most common female malignancy. It has been demonstrated that cervical screening programmes are associated with improved rate of cure of cervical cancer.

There are several risk factors associated with cervical cancer. The presence of the human papilloma virus (HPV) (highest risks are HPV types 16 and 18), women of low socioeconomic status, multiparous, those engaging in sexual activity at a young age or with multiple partners and cigarette smoking, all increase the risk. Women with a history of sexually transmitted infections, especially herpes or genital warts, and who do not attend cervical screening are also at greater risk. Those women who are immunosuppressed have a higher risk of cervical carcinoma.

Pathophysiology

There are three types of cervical cancer:
- Squamous cell cervical cancer is the most common
- Adenocarcinoma cervical cancer is less common
- Mixed cell

All are diagnosed and treated in a similar way and all three cause both pre-invasive and invasive disease.

HPV is seen as the vector that confers susceptibility to neoplastic conversion or directly incites transmutation to a malignant phenotype in some infected epithelial cells. Neoplastic transformation usually originates at the squamocolumnar junction of the cervix (see Figure 49.1). Varying degrees of cervical intra-epithelial neoplasia (CIN) exist; these are graded from 1 to 3 on the basis of increasing severity of the lesion (see Figure 49.2). Carcinoma *in situ* exists when all epithelial layers consist of neoplastic cells. It usually takes 10–20 years for intra-epithelial neoplasia to progress to invasive disease. Histologically many tumours exhibit squamous histology. Invasive cancer breaches the epithelial basement membrane at any point.

Cervical smears may be particularly effective in detecting pre-invasive or early-stage disease as women with early invasive cervix cancer may have a cervix that appears normal to the naked eye. The majority of these women are asymptomatic; however, with advanced cancer women often experience symptoms.

Invasive cancers display two chief modes of extension: local spread and metastasis via lymphatic system and bloodstream. Cervical cancer can have an ulcerative or exophytic appearance. Local expansion usually involves extension to the endocervix or vaginal fornices, followed by progressive infiltration of parametrial tissues, uterine corpus, bladder or rectum. Lymphatic dissemination usually occurs in a stepwise progression. Pelvic nodes become involved; spread via the bloodstream may give rise to distant implants of cancer in lungs, bones, liver or other tissue. The likelihood of metastasis grows with expanding size and expanse of tumour.

Signs and symptoms

Screening detects a substantial number of cases. The first symptoms of established cervical carcinoma include vaginal discharge, varying in amount, which is either intermittent or continuous. In the early stages bleeding can be spontaneous, but can occur after sex, micturition or defaecation. Women may ignore this if it is scanty and attribute this to normal menstrual dysfunction. On occasion, severe vaginal bleeding may require emergency hospital admission. There may be vaginal discomfort and urinary symptoms.

Late symptoms can include painless haematuria, chronic urinary frequency, painless fresh rectal bleeding, altered bowel habit, leg oedema, pain and hydronephrosis, leading to renal failure that may indicate late signs of pelvic wall involvement. In more advanced disease, women develop pelvic discomfort or poorly localized pain described as dull or boring in the suprapubic or sacral regions; this can be persistent or intermittent.

Examination can be relatively normal in early stage cancer. On the cervix there may be white or red patches. With progression of the disease this can lead to an abnormal appearance of the cervix and vagina, as a result of erosion, ulcer or tumour. There may be a mass or bleeding on rectal examination as a result of erosion. A pelvic bulkiness/mass may be present when bimanual palpation is undertaken, due to pelvic spread. Lymphatic or vascular obstruction can cause the development of leg oedema. With the presence of liver metastases there may be hepatomegaly. Pleural effusion or bronchial obstruction indicates pulmonary metastases.

Investigations

If cervical cancer is suspected, a number of investigations and tests are required to confirm diagnosis and to stage the disease. The following investigations may be undertaken. A colposcope is used to show the cervix in detail, acting as a magnifying glass to identify abnormal cervical cells. A biopsy is taken from the cervix and histologically examined. Large loop excision of the transformation zone (LLETZ) is used when the colposcope fails to identify any abnormality. Local anaesthesia is used and a thin wire, which is shaped in a loop, is then used to cut away the affected area. Needle excision of the transformation zone (NETZ) is similar to LLETZ. The thin wire used to cut away the affected area is straight, as opposed to a loop, acting like a knife permitting the precise area of affected tissue to excised.

Cone biopsy, used when the abnormal area in the cervix cannot be seen with a colposcope, is usually conducted under a general anaesthetic, although local anaesthetic can be used (see Figure 49.3).

Other investigations include full blood count, renal and liver function tests, chest X-ray, intravenous urogram, CT scan, barium enema or proctoscopy (to assess rectal involvement), cystoscopy (assesses bladder invasion) and MRI scan.

Management

The treatment of cancer of the cervix will depend on the stage. There are several approaches to treatment, for example surgery, radiotherapy, pharmacotherapy chemotherapy or a combination of these treatments. The extent of surgery will be dictated by the tumour stage, the age of the patient as well as any comorbidities. Normally, a combination of external beam therapy and intra-cavity brachytherapy is used.

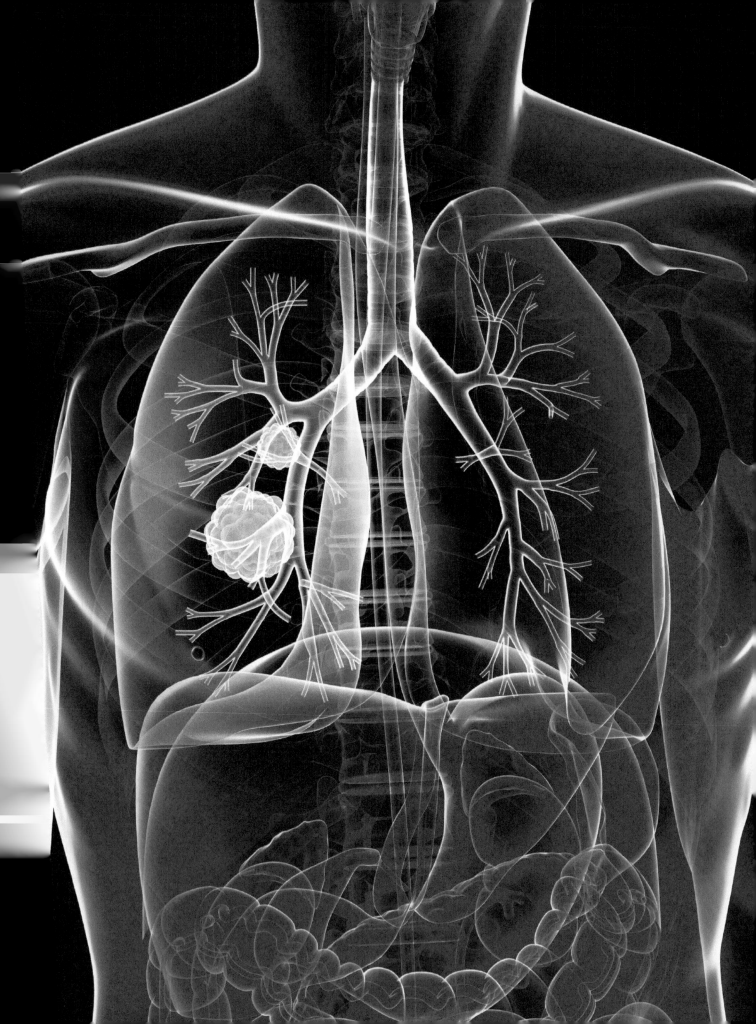

The adrenal glands

The adrenal glands are located at the superior poles of the two kidneys and are made up of two distinct parts, the adrenal medulla and adrenal cortex. The medulla acts with the central nervous system to secrete the hormones epinephrine and norepinephrine in response to sympathetic stimulation. The adrenal cortex is anatomically separated into three zones: zona glomerulosa, zona fasciculata, and zona reticularis. The outer zona glomerulosa is responsible for secreting the aldosterone (a mineralo-corticoid) and the inner zonae fasciculate and reticularis, responsible for secreting glucocorticoids (e.g. cortisol) and androgens. See Figure 51.1.

An adrenocorticotropic hormone (ACTH), stimulates the adrenal cortex to synthesize and secrete cortisol, which regulates carbohydrate, protein and lipid metabolism, and aldosterone, which regulates fluid and electrolyte balance through sodium and potassium homeostasis. The adrenal cortex also secretes other steroids with glucocorticoid, mineralo-corticoid, or both activities, but in much smaller quantities.

Pathophysiology

When there is a reduction in the output of adrenal hormones, for example glucocorticoids and/or mineralo-corticoids, this is termed as adrenal insufficiency. There are two kinds of adrenal insufficiency. Primary insufficiency is an inability of the adrenal glands to produce sufficient steroid hormones to meet physiological needs, despite release of ACTH from the pituitary (Addison's disease is the name given to the autoimmune cause of this insufficiency). Glucocorticoid and often mineralo-corticoid hormones are lost. Secondary insufficiency is inadequate pituitary or hypothalamic stimulation of the adrenal glands. Secondary adrenocortical insufficiency happens when exogenous steroids have suppressed the hypothalamic-pituitary-adrenal (HPA) axis. Too rapid withdrawal of exogenous steroid may precipitate adrenal crisis, or sudden stress may induce cortisol requirements in excess of the adrenal glands' ability to respond immediately.

Signs and symptoms

The signs and symptoms of adrenal insufficiency often develop gradually and these can include:

- Severe fatigue and weakness
- Increased pigmentation of the skin
- Syncope and hypotension, with orthostatic hypostension
- Anorexia, nausea, vomiting, diarrhoea
- Salt craving (hyponatraemia)
- Myalgia and arthralgia
- Depression
- Altered menstrual cycles

As a result of the sometimes non-specific nature of symptoms and their gradual progression, they are often missed or ignored until a relatively minor infection results in an abnormally long recovery, prompting an investigation. Often, it is not until a crisis is triggered that attention is turned to the adrenal glands.

Investigations

A detailed history and physical examination are needed. The signs and symptoms associated with adrenal insufficiency, for example exhaustion, fatigue, muscle weakness and weight loss, are often unclear. Adrenal insufficiency can cause changes in the serum sodium (hyponatraemia) and high serum potassium (hyperkalaemia). There may also be anaemia. These findings are somewhat general and can be found in the context of a number of conditions other than adrenal insufficiency.

To establish a diagnosis, a short synacthen test (SST) has to be performed. This test is also called ACTH stimulation test or a cosyntropin test. The SST determines the ability of the adrenal glands to produce cortisol in response to ACTH (the pituitary hormone regulating adrenal cortisol production). When the test is undertaken a baseline blood sample is drawn prior to injecting a dose of ACTH, followed by drawing of a second sample of blood 30–60 minutes after the ACTH injection. If the adrenal glands are functioning, cortisol production in the second sample exceeds a particular level, (usually 500–550 nmol/L). Adrenal glands that are poorly functioning will not be able to produce this amount of cortisol.

Other investigations may include electrocardiograph, abdominal X-ray, CT scan or MRI of adrenals, and 24-hour urine test to assess alterations in the biosynthesis of adrenal cortical hormones. Abnormal findings in adrenal insufficiency can be found in Figure 51.2.

Management

Adrenal crisis can occur after physical or mental stress. This could be life threatening and is characterized by volume depletion, hypotension and vascular collapse. When a patient is suspected of suffering from adrenal insufficiency and concurrently shows signs of possible adrenal crisis (persistent vomiting with profound muscle weakness, hypotension or even shock, extreme sleepiness or even coma), admission to hospital as an emergency is needed. Emergency treatment should be initiated without delay as the diagnosis can still be formally confirmed later by the short synacthen test once the patient is stable again.

Only those who have been conclusively diagnosed with adrenal insufficiency should receive adrenal hormone replacement therapy as advised by an endocrinologist. A normal adrenal gland does not need supplements to function effectively, either the adrenal is working effectively and requires no treatment or there is insufficiency due to adrenal or pituitary failure, as measured by an endocrinologist.

The person should be provided with information about the condition, advised to wear a medical alert type bracelet and should carry a steroid card. During intercurrent illness, if the patient is tolerating oral medication, the dose should be doubled until recovered. If the patient is unwell and unable to take oral medication then it should be given parenterally; they will need to be given intramuscular hydrocortisone and be taught how to administer it.

For glucocorticoid replacement, hydrocortisone is the mainstay of treatment. Secondary adrenocortical insufficiency may involve multiple deficiencies, that is, panhypopituitarism. Other causes include ACTH suppression by sodium valporate, metastases, craniopharyngioma, tuberculosis, postpartum pituitary necrosis, trauma and following radiotherapy or surgery. Hormone replacement therapy may be required with more definitive treatment, for example surgical removal of a pituitary tumour.

52 Cushing's syndrome

Figure 52.1   Cushing's syndrome

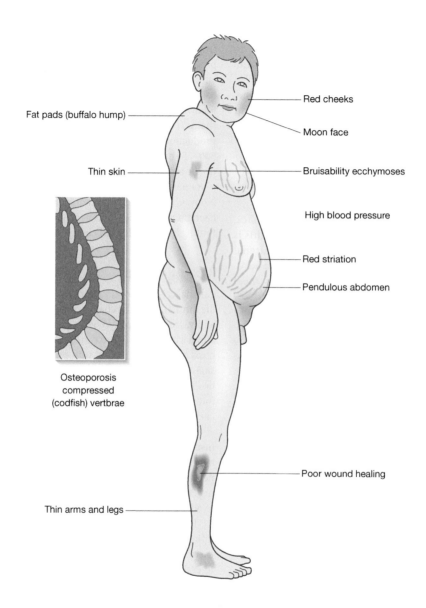

Fat pads (buffalo hump)

Thin skin

Red cheeks

Moon face

Bruisability ecchymoses

High blood pressure

Red striation

Pendulous abdomen

Osteoporosis
compressed
(codfish) vertbrae

Poor wound healing

Thin arms and legs

Pathophysiology for Nurses at a Glance, First Edition. Muralitharan Nair and Ian Peate. © 2015 John Wiley & Sons, Ltd. Published 2015 by John Wiley & Sons, Ltd.
Companion website: www.ataglanceseries.com/nursing/pathophysiology

The musculoskeletal system

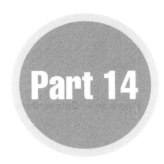

Part 14

Chapters

54 Osteoarthritis

Figure 54.1 Osteoarthritis

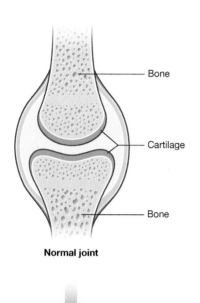

Normal joint

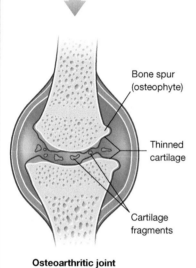

Osteoarthritic joint

Figure 54.2 Classification of joints

Type of joint	Examples	Structure
Hinge	Elbow, knee	
Pivot	Radius and ulna, the atlas and axis	
Ball and socket	Hip, shoulder	
Saddle	The carpometacarpal joints of the thumb	
Condyloid	The radiocarpal and metacarpophalangeal joints of the hand	
Gliding	Intertarsal and intercarpal joints of the hands and feet	

Source:
Peate, Wild & Nair,
Nursing Practice:
Knowledge and Care, 2014

Pathophysiology for Nurses at a Glance, First Edition. Muralitharan Nair and Ian Peate. © 2015 John Wiley & Sons, Ltd. Published 2015 by John Wiley & Sons, Ltd.
Companion website: www.ataglanceseries.com/nursing/pathophysiology

Osteoarthritis

Osteoarthritis is the most common type of joint disease. It is a degenerative disorder arising from the biochemical breakdown of articular (hyaline) cartilage in the synovial joints. It is characterized by loss of articular (the joint) cartilage as well as an abnormal growth of new bone (bone spur). Osteoarthritis involves not only the articular cartilage but also the entire joint organ, including the subchondral bone and synovium (see Figure 54.1).

Joints can be classified in functional or structural terms. Functional classifications, based on movement are synarthroses (immovable), amphiarthroses (slightly moveable) and diarthroses (freely moveable). A structural classification categorizes joints as synovial, fibrous and cartilaginous. See Figure 54.2.

Normal synovial joints allow a significant amount of motion along their extremely smooth articular surface. These joints are composed of an articular cartilage, subchondral bone, synovial membrane, synovial fluid and joint capsule. The normal articular surface of synovial joints consists of articular cartilage (composed of chondrocytes) enclosed by an extracellular matrix that includes various macromolecules, most importantly proteoglycans and collagen. The cartilage enables joint function, protecting the underlying subchondral bone by distributing large loads, maintaining low contact stresses, as well as reducing friction at the joint.

Synovial fluid is formed through a serum ultrafiltration process by cells forming the synovial membrane (synoviocytes). Hyaluronic acid (HA, known also as hyaluronate) is also produced by the synovial cells, a glycosaminoglycan that is the major non-cellular component of synovial fluid. Synovial fluid brings nutrients to the avascular articular cartilage, as well as providing the viscosity required to absorb shock from slow movements, as well as the elasticity needed to absorb shock as a result of rapid movements.

Pathophysiology

This degenerative disease affects the whole joint, any joint can be affected. However, osteoarthritis most commonly affects the knees, hips, hands, neck and low back. It usually affects multiple joints but it can be isolated to one joint. It can lead to significant problems with mobility as well as having socioeconomic and psychosocial ramifications.

There are a number of risk factors for osteoarthritis and these include increasing age, obesity, trauma, family history (genetics), decreased levels of sex hormones, myalgia, repetitive use, infection, crystal deposition, acromegaly, previous inflammatory arthritis, heritable metabolic causes, haemoglobinopathies, neuropathic disorders, disorders of bone, previous surgical procedures (e.g. meniscectomy).

Pathologically in osteoarthritis, there are focal areas of damage to load-bearing articular cartilage, new bone formation at the joint margins (osteophytosis), alteration in the subchondral bone (sclerosis), inflammation of the synovium (synovitis) and thickening of the joint capsule. Osteoarthritis can be seen as a continuum of the normal repair process that occurs in all joint tissues as a result of joint trauma. In some people, however, it may be due to severe trauma or problems with the repair process; there is continued tissue damage with the result of symptomatic osteoarthritis.

Conventionally, osteoarthritis was believed to affect primarily the articular cartilage of synovial joints; however, pathophysiological evidence now demonstrates changes occurring in the synovial fluid, as well as in the underlying (subchondral) bone, the overlying joint capsule and other joint tissues.

Osteoarthritis has been classified as a non-inflammatory arthritis, yet increasing evidence demonstrates that inflammation occurs as cytokines and metalloproteinases are released into the joint. These agents are involved in the excessive matrix degradation that characterizes cartilage degeneration in osteoarthritis.

In early osteoarthritis, swelling of the cartilage frequently occurs, reflecting an effort by the chondrocytes to repair cartilage damage. This may last for years or decades and is depicted by hypertrophic repair of the articular cartilage.

As the condition develops, the levels of proteoglycans finally drop to very low levels, causing the cartilage to soften, with a loss of elasticity compromising joint surface integrity further. Microscopically, flaking and fibrillations (vertical clefts) develop along the usually smooth articular cartilage on the surface of an osteoarthritic joint. Loss of cartilage results in loss of joint space as time progresses.

Erosion of damaged cartilage in an osteoarthritic joint progresses until there is exposure of underlying cartilage and the protective cartilage continues to articulate with the opposing surface.

The damaged subchondral bone can also undergo cystic degeneration. Osteoarthritic cysts are also referred to as subchondral cysts, pseudocysts, or geodes. Fragmentation of these osteophytes or of the articular cartilage itself results in the presence of intra-articular loose bodies.

Signs and symptoms

The progression of osteoarthritis is typically slow, occurring over several years or decades. The patient can become less and less active, and more susceptible to morbidities related to decreasing physical activity. Structural changes can often occur, with no accompanying symptoms, but joints may appear normal.

Pain is often the first source of morbidity, described as being deep, achy joint pain exacerbated by extensive use; there may be a reduced range of movement and crepitus. Stiffness during rest can develop, along with morning joint stiffness. In the beginning pain can be relieved by rest and responds to simple analgesia. Pain may become more evident even during rest and not respond to medications. There may be joint swelling/synovitis, periarticular tenderness, bony swelling and deformity, and muscle weakness/wasting around the affected joint.

Investigations

Diagnosis is typically based on clinical examination. When disease is advanced it can be seen on plain X-rays. MRI may be useful to distinguish other causes of joint pain. For swollen joints joint aspiration may be considered.

Management

The goals of treatment include alleviation of pain and improvement of functional status. Patients should receive a combination of non-pharmacological and pharmacological treatment. National guidelines are available.

55 Osteoporosis

Figure 55.1 A healthy and an osteoporotic bone

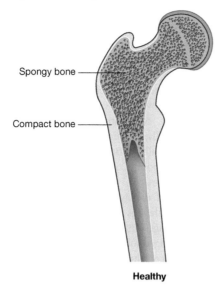

Spongy bone

Compact bone

Healthy

Osteoporosis

Table 55.1 Risk factors

• Increasing age	• Corticosteroid therapy	• Anorexia nervosa	• Primary hyperparathyroidism
• Reduced BMD	• Cushing's syndrome	• Poor diet (calcium-deficient)	• Hyperthyroidism
• Parental history of hip fracture	• Ankylosing spondylitis	• Malabsorption syndromes (coeliac disease)	• Osteogenesis imperfeceta
• Four or more units of alcohol daily	• Crohn's disease	• Prolonged immobilization	• Caucasian or Asian origin
• Rheumatoid arthritis	• Untreated premature menopause or prolonged secondary amenorrhoea	• Smoking	• Post-transplantation
• Female gender	• Low body mass (<19 kg/m^2)	• Primary hypogonadism (men and women)	• Chronic renal failure

Figure 55.2 Osteoporosis

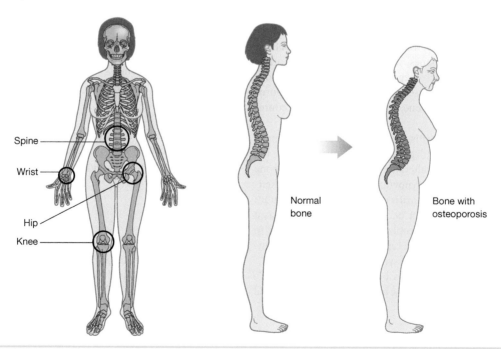

Spine

Wrist

Hip

Knee

Normal bone

Bone with osteoporosis

Pathophysiology for Nurses at a Glance, First Edition. Muralitharan Nair and Ian Peate. © 2015 John Wiley & Sons, Ltd. Published 2015 by John Wiley & Sons, Ltd.
Companion website: www.ataglanceseries.com/nursing/pathophysiology

Gout

This is an acute joint disease, an inflammatory arthropathy, an arthritis, resulting in acute inflammatory state and subsequent tissue damage. This is a very painful condition. It causes a spectrum of disease.

Pathophysiology

Gout is a disorder of metabolism permitting uric acid or urate to accumulate in blood and tissues; when supersaturated urate salts precipitate forming needlelike crystals, these are less soluble under acid conditions and at low temperatures, as occurring in cool, peripheral joints of the metatarsophalangeal joint of the big toe) (see Figure 57.1).

Gout can be classified into primary or secondary gout subject to the cause of hyperuricaemia. Primary gout occurs predominantly in males aged 30–60 years who present with acute attacks. Secondary gout is quite often due to chronic diuretic therapy. It occurs in older people and is often associated with osteoarthritis.

Gout affects the upper and lower limbs, with acute attacks. It can present with painful, tophaceous deposits (there may be discharge) in Heberden's and Bouchard's nodes.

The majority of people with hyperuricaemia never develop gout and gouty patients may not have hyperuricaemia at presentation. Most patients (about 90%) with gout develop excess urate as a result of an inability to excrete adequate amounts of uric acid in the urine. Most of the remaining patients either over consume purines or produce excessive amounts of uric acid endogenously (overproduction).

Most cases of primary gout are due to under-secretion of uric acid. Fewer than 10% of cases are as a result of overproduction. Many conditions and medications have been associated with an increase in plasma urate levels, especially metabolic syndrome. A genetic predisposition for hyperuricaemia exists; except in rare genetic disorders, however, the development of gout in people who are hyperuricaemic is mediated by environmental factors.

Overproduction of uric acid occurs in disorders that cause high cell turnover, releasing purines present in high concentration in cell nuclei. Cell lysis from chemotherapy can elevate uric acid levels, as can excessive exercise and obesity. Causes of secondary gout due to under excretion of uric acid include renal insufficiency, starvation or dehydration, some drugs and chronic abuse of alcohol (particularly beer and spirits).

The development of gout occurs where there are excessive stores of uric acid in the form of monosodium urate. Uric acid is an end-stage by-product of purine metabolism, which is usually removed by renal excretion. If excretion is ineffective in maintaining serum urate levels below the saturation level of 6.8 mg/dL, hyperuricaemia may develop. The presence of urate crystals in the soft tissues and synovial tissues is a requirement for a gout attack. These crystals can also be found in synovial fluid or on the cartilage surface in the absence of joint inflammation (see Figure 57.2).

A gout attack may be triggered by release of crystals (e.g. from partial dissolution of a micro tophus caused by changing serum urate levels) or precipitation of crystals in a supersaturated microenvironment. In either situation urate crystals interact with intracellular and surface receptors of local dendritic cells and macrophages, triggering a danger signal activating the innate immune system, leading to inflammatory mediator production.

There are several risk factors (comorbid conditions) associated with a higher incidence of gout: hypertension, diabetes mellitus, renal insufficiency, hypertriglyceridaemia, hypercholesterolaemia, obesity, anaemia. Foods rich in purines: anchovies, sardines, sweetbreads, kidney, liver and meat extracts, consumption of fructose-rich foods and beverages are associated with an increased risk of gout. There is evidence that there may be a genetic link to gout.

The pathophysiology, clinical presentation and acute-phase treatment of gout and pseudogout are similar; however, the underlying causes of the diseases are very different. Many cases of pseudogout in the elderly are idiopathic. Pseudogout has been linked with trauma and a variety of metabolic abnormalities, for example hyperparathyroidism and haemochromatosis.

Risk factors for pseudogout include use of loop diuretics and proton pump inhibitors. Pseudogout has an underlying genetic component, comorbid conditions (e.g. osteoarthritis) and environmental factors may play a much stronger role.

Signs and symptoms

The development of acute pain in a joint that has become swollen, tender and erythematous and which reaches its climax over a 6–12 hour period is highly suggestive of crystal arthropathy, though not specifically of gout. Inflammation reaches its peak within 24 hours, often with fever and malaise. Some people may only present with connective tissue tophi.

There is evidence of synovitis and swelling and extreme tenderness with overlying erythema. Atypical attacks can occur, with tenosynovitis, bursitis and cellulitis lasting one or two days. There may be irregular firm nodules mainly around extensor surfaces of fingers, hands, forearms, elbows, Achilles tendons and ear, in chronic tophaceous gout. Tophi are asymmetrical with a chalky appearance under the skin.

Investigations

National guidelines are available that recommend investigations. A clinical diagnosis can be made with reasonable accuracy with typical presentations such as: inflammation of the first metatarsophalangeal joint (known also as podagra) with hyperuricaemia; presence of monosodium urate crystals in synovial fluid or tophi; Gram staining and culture of synovial fluid. Serum uric acid levels should be estimated but as a diagnostic tool this is limited. Renal uric acid secretion (24-hour urine sample is needed) may be helpful in diagnosis. Radiographs may be useful in chronic gout. CT scanning can help in less accessible areas.

Management

Pain relief is a priority. The objective is to relieve pain and inflammation as quickly as possible. Rest and an ice pack may be useful; elevate the joint and avoid trauma. Non-steroidal anti-inflammatory drugs, colchicine and corticosteroids can help with pain and inflammation. Lifestyle issues such as weight loss, exercise, diet, alcohol consumption and fluid intake should be discussed.

Figure 57.3 shows the complications of gout.

58 **Rheumatoid arthritis**

Figure 58.1   Rheumatoid arthritis

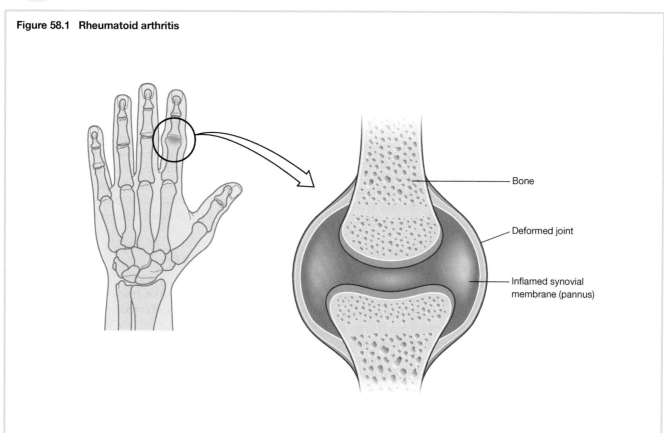

Rheumatoid arthritis (RA) is a chronic systemic inflammatory disease with an unknown cause. An external trigger, for example cigarette smoking, infection or trauma triggers an autoimmune reaction, causing synovial hypertrophy and chronic joint inflammation, with the possibility for extra-articular manifestations; the condition is thought to occur in genetically susceptible people. Early diagnosis of RA and effective treatment with drugs that reduce joint destruction and disability (disease-modifying anti-rheumatic drugs (DMRADs)) is essential. When mechanical damage has occurred, pain and joint deformity usually necessitates use of aids and appliances; eventually surgery is needed.

The condition affects the hands and feet, though any joint lined by a synovial membrane may be involved. Extra-articular involvement of organs such as the skin, heart, lungs and eyes can be significant.

Rheumatoid arthritis

While inflammation of the tissue surrounding the joints and inflammatory arthritis are typical features of rheumatoid arthritis, the disease can also cause inflammation and injury in other organs in the body. Autoimmune diseases occur when the body's tissues are mistakenly attacked by their own immune system. The immune system contains a complex organization of cells and antibodies that seek and destroy invaders of the body, particularly infections. Those with autoimmune diseases have antibodies in their blood that target their own body tissues, where they can be associated with inflammation.

The rheumatoid factor is an antibody that is detectable in the blood of 80% of adults with rheumatoid arthritis. Rheumatoid factor can be detected in the blood of normal people and of those with other autoimmune diseases that are not rheumatoid arthritis. In those with rheumatoid arthritis, high levels of rheumatoid factor can indicate a tendency towards more aggressive disease and/or a tendency to develop rheumatoid nodules and rheumatoid lung disease.

There is no known cure for rheumatoid arthritis.

Pathophysiology

Women are more likely to develop RA than men and the peak incidence occurs when the person is in their forties or fifties. The connective tissue that is usually destroyed first is the lining of the joints, the synovial membrane. The inflammation becomes unremitting and then it spreads to the surrounding structures of the joint – the articular cartilage and the fibrous joint capsule. The ligaments and the tendons will eventually become inflamed. The pathogenesis of RA is not completely understood, synovial cell hyperplasia and endothelial cell activation are early events in the pathological process that progresses to uncontrolled inflammation and resultant cartilage and bone destruction (see Figure 58.1). The inflammation is distinguished by the accumulation of white blood cells, complement activation, extensive phagocytosis and scarring. Unlike other types of arthritis, RA occurs in symmetrical pattern. Genetic factors and immune system abnormalities contribute to disease propagation.

CD4 T cells, mononuclear phagocytes, fibroblasts, osteoclasts and neutrophils play key cellular roles in the pathophysiology of RA, whereas B cells produce autoantibodies (i.e. RFs). Abnormal production of numerous cytokines, chemokines and other inflammatory mediators have been established in people with RA. Inflammation and vigorous proliferation of the synovium (pannus) leads to destruction of several tissues, including cartilage, bone, tendons, ligaments and blood vessels. These processes slowly destroy bone, causing much pain and deformity.

Signs and symptoms

The characteristic feature of RA is persistent symmetric polyarthritis (synovitis) affecting the hands and feet; however, any joint lined by a synovial membrane may be involved. RA severity can vary over time; chronic RA results in the progressive development of various degrees of joint destruction, deformity and a significant decline in functional status. Extra-articular involvement of organs such as the skin, heart, lungs and eyes can also be significant. There may be fatigue, malaise, morning stiffness, weight loss and low-grade pyrexia.

The onset of RA is insidious, beginning with systemic features such as fever, malaise, arthralgia and weakness, which can occur prior to the overt appearance of joint inflammation and swelling. The person may experience difficulty in performing activities of living.

Investigations

Diagnosis is essentially clinical; investigations are important in assessment and exclusion of other possible diagnoses. Non-specific investigations include full blood count, C-reactive protein and plasma viscosity, liver function tests, antinuclear antibody, uric acid/synovial fluid analysis. National guidance exists concerning other investigations, for example rheumatoid factor, and anti-cyclic citrullinated peptide antibodies if the patient is negative for rheumatoid factor. Radiography remains the first choice for imaging in RA, with X-ray of the hands and feet.

Management

The goals of treatment include:
- Pain relief and reduction of swelling
- Prevention of structural damage
- Preservation of function

Administration of analgesia NSAIDs; cyclo-oxygenase-2 (COX-2) inhibitors; non-drug management options, such as transcutaneous electrical nerve stimulation may help; drugs to suppress neuropathic pain such as carbamazepine or amitriptyline, may also be of value. The inflamed joints should be rested during exacerbations, with rest periods each day, the use of alternating hot and cold packs, occupational therapy and physiotherapy. Low-dose oral corticosteroids can be used in combination with disease-modifying anti-rheumatic drugs (DMARDs) for short-term relief of signs and symptoms and in the medium to long term to reduce radiological damage. DMARDs (methotrexate and sulfasalazine) either affect the immune response or suppress the disease process and improve the symptoms and signs of the arthritis; they may also improve the extra-articular manifestations such as vasculitis, in addition to exerting systemic effects. Biological therapies have been shown to be effective in the treatment of RA.

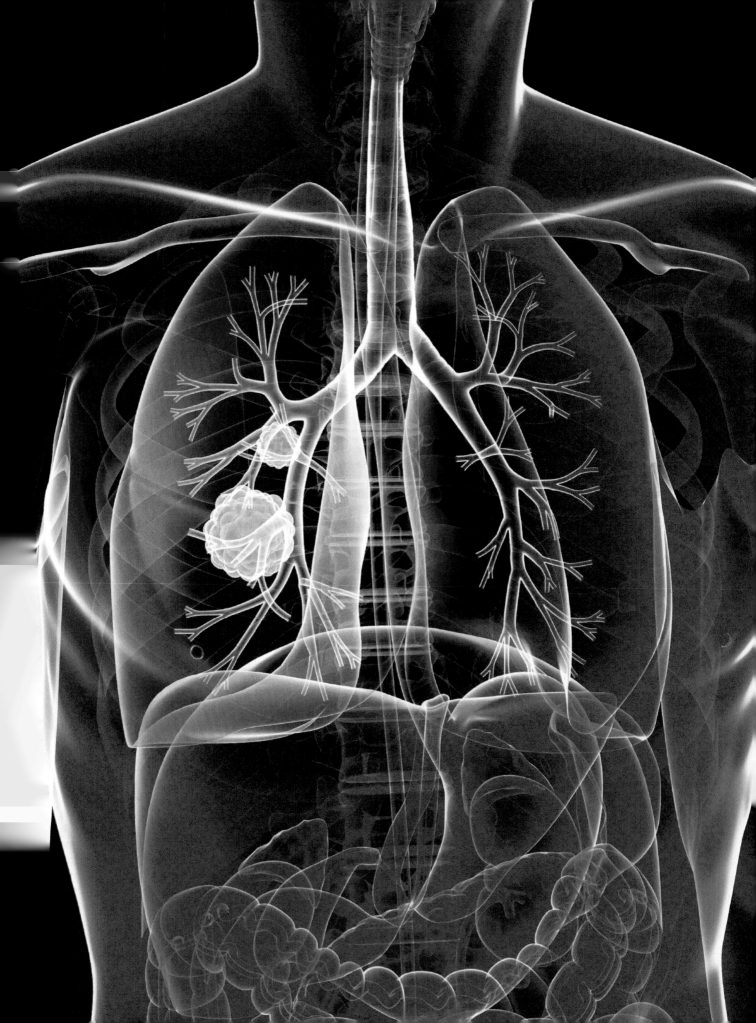

Psoriasis

Psoriasis (also called psoriasis vulgaris) is a common skin condition that is characterized by focal formation of inflamed, raised plaques that constantly shed scales, resulting from excessive growth of skin epithelial cells. It is a T-lymphocyte mediated autoimmune disease. Psoriasis is a complex, chronic, multifactorial, inflammatory disease involving hyperproliferation of the keratinocytes in the epidermis, with an increase in the epidermal cell turnover rate (6–9 times faster than normal). Environmental, genetic and immunological factors seem to play a role. T cells are induced to produce cytokines, which stimulate keratinocyte proliferation and the production of dermal antigenic adhesion molecules in the local blood vessels, further stimulating the T-cell cytokine response. The disease most commonly manifests on the skin of the elbows, knees, scalp, lumbosacral areas, intergluteal clefts and glans penis (see Figure 60.1).

The prevalence of psoriasis is likely to be about 1.3–2.2% in the UK, with highest prevalence in white people. It can occur at any age, but first presentation is usually before the age of 35 years. It is uncommon in children. The majority of people have plaque psoriasis. Joint disease is associated with psoriasis in a significant proportion of patients.

The condition is classified as mild if less than 2% of the body surface area is affected; if 2–10% of the body surface is affected this is said to be moderate and if more than 10% it is severe.

Psoriasis is a chronic, non-contagious, multisystem, inflammatory disorder. Psoriasis has a tendency to wax and wane, with flares related to systemic or environmental factors, including life stress events and infection. It impacts heavily on quality of life and potentially long-term survival.

Pathophysiology

Multiple types of psoriasis have been identified, with plaque-type psoriasis, also known as discoid psoriasis, being the most common type. Plaque psoriasis usually presents with plaques on the scalp, trunk and limbs. These plaques appear as focal, raised, inflamed, oedematous lesions covered with silvery-white 'micaceous' scales'.

Types of psoriasis include plaque (the most common), guttate, inverse, erythrodermic, pustular and psoriatic arthritis.

There are a number of risk factors associated with psoriasis. There is a genetic tendency to develop psoriasis with a multifactorial pattern of inheritance. Environmental factors may trigger or exacerbate plaque psoriasis, including sunlight; there is a decrease in severity during periods of increased sun exposure but a small minority have an aggravation of symptoms during strong sunlight and sunburn. Streptococcal infection is associated with the development of guttate psoriasis, but this can also apply to chronic plaque psoriasis. Psychological stress can play a role. Hormonal changes (e.g. in the postpartum period) may exacerbate psoriasis. Some drugs can trigger psoriasis, as can smoking and alcohol. Psoriasis may be spread to uninvolved skin by various types of trauma.

The pathogenesis of the condition is not fully understood. Triggers can bring on an infectious episode, such as traumatic insult and stressful life event. In many people, no obvious trigger exists at all. Once triggered, however, there is substantial leukocyte recruitment to the dermis and epidermis that causes the characteristic psoriatic plaques. See Figure 60.2 Normal skin and psoriasis.

The epidermis becomes infiltrated by large numbers of activated T cells, capable of inducing keratinocyte proliferation. Ultimately, a ramped-up, deregulated inflammatory process occurs, with a large production of various cytokines. Many of the clinical features of psoriasis are explained by the large production of such mediators.

Key findings in the affected skin of patients with psoriasis include vascular engorgement as a result of superficial blood vessel dilation and altered epidermal cell cycle. Epidermal hyperplasia leads to an accelerated cell turnover, leading to improper cell maturation.

Cells that usually lose their nuclei in the stratum granulosum preserve their nuclei; this is known as parakeratosis. In addition to parakeratosis, affected epidermal cells fail to release adequate levels of lipids, which normally cement adhesions of corneocytes. As a result, poorly adherent stratum corneum is formed, leading to the flaking, scaly presentation of psoriasis lesions; the surface often resembles silver scales.

Signs and symptoms

In plaque-type erythematous plaques with slivery scales, symmetrical involvement, can be pruritic and painful, often appearing at areas of epidermal injury. Guttate appears as individual red drop-like patterns occurring on the trunk, arms or legs, not as thick as plaque psoriasis. Inverse, bright red patches that are smooth and shiny, affect flexural areas such as the axilla and groin. There is erythrodermic, redness over most of the body, a scalded-like appearance, with severe pruritus and signs of systemic illness. Pustular blisters containing purulent non-infective material surrounded by red skin on the palms and the soles, or on widespread areas, may be seen mainly in adults and is exacerbated by the sun. Psoriatic arthritis is associated with joint pain, accompanying skin involvement.

Investigations

History and physical examination will determine diagnosis. It is unusual for a skin biopsy to be used to confirm diagnosis.

Management

The severity of the disease determines treatment. It is essential to offer a full explanation of psoriasis, including reassurance that the condition is neither infectious nor malignant.

Management includes, first-line therapy with topical therapies such as corticosteroids, vitamin D analogues, dithranol and tar preparations. Second-line therapy includes phototherapy, broad-band or narrow-band ultraviolet B light, application of complex topical therapies such as dithranol in Lassar's paste or crude coal tar and photochemotherapy, psoralens in combination with UVA irradiation (PUVA) and non-biological systemic agents. Third-line therapy refers to systemic biological therapies.

Regular use of emollients reduces scale and itching. During a flare-up of psoriatic arthritis the joint should be rested. Wrist splints, footwear, gentle massage or applying heat may help. NSAIDs ease pain and stiffness. Intra-articular steroid therapy reduces inflammation. Disease-modifying anti-rheumatic drugs aim to suppress inflammation, reducing the damaging effect of the disease on the joints. The person should be encouraged to keep as active as possible. Surgery to replace joints may be needed.

61 Acne vulgaris

Figure 61.1 A pilosebaceous unit

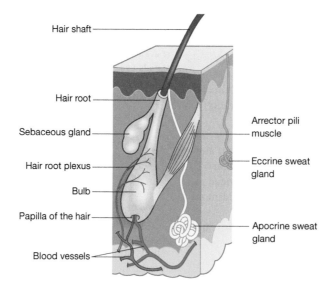

Hair shaft

Hair root

Sebaceous gland

Hair root plexus

Bulb

Papilla of the hair

Blood vessels

Arrector pili muscle

Eccrine sweat gland

Apocrine sweat gland

Source:
Peate, Wild & Nair, *Nursing Practice: Knowledge and Care*, 2014

Figure 61.2 The pathogenesis of acne

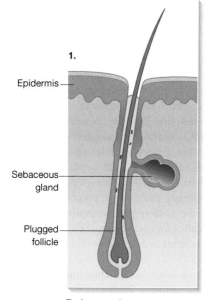
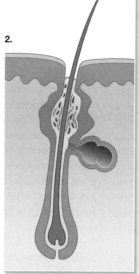
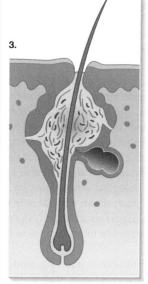
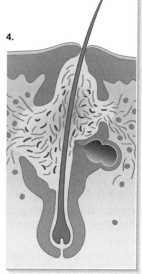

Epidermis

Sebaceous gland

Plugged follicle

1.

Early comedone
- Accumulation of epithelial cells and keratin

2.

Later comedone
- Accumulation of shed keratin and sebum

3.

Inflammatory papule/pustule
- Propionibacterium acnes proliferation
- Mild inflammation

4.

Nodule cyst
- Marked inflammation
- Scarring

Acne vulgaris

Acne vulgaris is a common skin condition that affects most people in the UK at some time in their lives. It is a disorder of the pilosebaceous follicles; the areas of skin with the densest population of sebaceous follicles include the face, the upper part of the chest and the back (see Figure 61.1).

At puberty androgens increase the production of sebum from enlarged sebaceous glands that become blocked and infected with *Propionibacterium acnes* causing an inflammatory reaction. Comedones (follicles impacted and distended by incompletely desquamated keratinocytes and sebum) may be open (blackheads) or closed (whiteheads). Inflammation leads to papules, pustules and nodules.

Just under a quarter of people with acne will have severe acne; this can cause severe psychological problems, undermining self-assurance and self-esteem at a vulnerable time in the person's life.

Most teenagers can expect to experience acne of some degree during the adolescent years. Genetic factors play a part and a positive family history is usually a factor, concordance among twins has been demonstrated. The condition affects boys more than girls and usually happens in adolescence, when hormones are in a state of change. In girls it may flare up when they are premenstrual, it can also be associated with polycystic ovarian syndrome. It can come about as the result of abnormal production of androgens. This can occur in testosterone replacement therapy, abuse of anabolic steroids, Cushing's disease or in virilizing tumours in women, such as arrhenoblastoma.

Pathophysiology

The pathogenesis of acne vulgaris is multifactorial. The significant factor is genetics. Acne develops as a result of an interplay of the following four factors: (1) follicular epidermal hyperproliferation with subsequent plugging of the follicle, (2) excess sebum production, (3) the presence and activity of the commensal bacteria *Propionibacterium acnes,* and (4) inflammation (see Figure 61.2).

Retention hyperkeratosis is the first recognized event in the development of acne vulgaris. The exact underlying cause of this hyperproliferation is unknown.

Androgen hormones (testosterone) have been implicated as the initial trigger. Comedones, which is the clinical lesion resulting from follicular plugging, begin to appear around sexual maturation (adrenarche) in those with acne in the T-zone area. The degree of comedonal acne in prepubertal girls correlates with circulating levels of the adrenal androgen dehydroepiandrosterone sulfate (DHEA-S). Furthermore, androgen hormone receptors are present in sebaceous glands; those people with malfunctioning androgen receptors do not develop acne.

Excess sebum is another significant factor in the development of acne vulgaris. Sebum production and excretion are controlled by a variety of different hormones and mediators. Androgen hormones in particular promote sebum production and release. Yet, most men and women with acne have normal circulating levels of androgen hormones. Androgen hormones are not the only regulators of the human sebaceous gland. There are other agents, for example growth hormone and insulin-like growth factor, also regulate the sebaceous gland and contribute to the development of acne

P acnes is an anaerobic organism that is present in acne lesions. The presence of *P acnes* encourages inflammation through a number of ways. *P acnes* stimulates inflammation producing pro-inflammatory mediators that diffuse through the wall of the follicle. *P acnes* activates on monocytes and neutrophils. Activation leads to the production of multiple pro-inflammatory cytokines, including interleukins 12 and 8 and tumour necrosis factor. Hypersensitivity to *P acnes* could also explain why some people develop inflammatory acne vulgaris and others do not.

Signs and symptoms

The condition is characterized by non-inflammatory, open or closed comedones and by inflammatory papules, pustules and nodules; the person usually has greasy skin. Local symptoms may include pain or tenderness. There are usually no systemic symptoms in acne vulgaris. Severe acne with associated systemic signs and symptoms, such as fever, is referred to as acne fulminans. Severe acne, characterized by multiple comedones, without the presence of systemic symptoms, is called acne conglobata. This severe form of acne frequently heals with disfiguring scars.

Investigations

There are usually no investigations required to make a diagnosis. Occasionally if investigations are required this is to explore a possible underlying cause, such as a virilizing tumour. Skin lesion culture may be necessary in those who do not respond to treatment, this is to exclude Gram negative folliculitis.

Management

The condition is usually mild and self-limiting. The face should be kept clean, and washed twice a day with soap and water. Branded antiseptic products may help. Use of the 1450-nm laser promotes improvement in acne. Blue light phototherapy can be useful for mild-to-moderate papulopustular acne. Topical preparations need to be applied to all affected areas and not only to existing lesions. Salicylic acid 10% has similar actions to retinoids. For mild papulopustular acne, benzoyl peroxide reduces production of sebum and comedones, inhibiting the growth of *P. acnes*. Topical erythromycin, clindamycin and tetracycline can be effective. Local treatment with topical retinoids such as isotretinoin, tretinoin or adapalene reduces comedones and has an anti-inflammatory effect. Systemic treatment can take several months to show any improvement; if tolerated it should be continued for 3–4 months and this may be combined with topical treatment. No specific oral antibiotic demonstrates superiority with respect to efficacy, tolerability or safety. Anti-androgen treatment, predominantly oestrogenic oral contraceptive, is an effective treatment for acne.

If scarring requires treatment then laser resurfacing, dermabrasion and chemical peels are used. Microdermabrasion is a simple outpatient procedure in which aluminum oxide crystals or other abrasive substances are blown on to the face and then vacuumed off.

62 Malignant melanoma

Figure 62.1 The location of a melanocyte

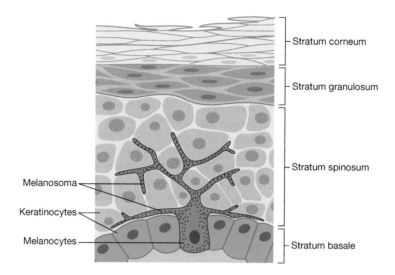

Figure 62.2 Melanocytes and exposure to UV radiation

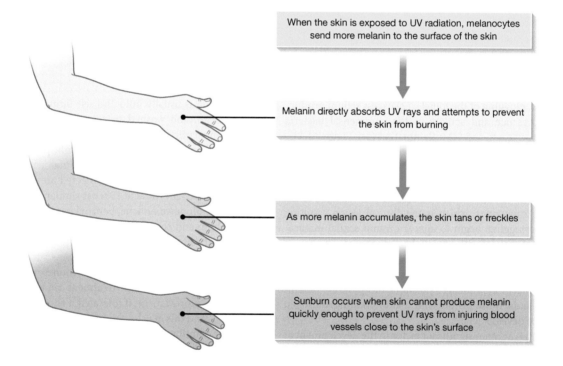

Table 62.1 The ABCDs for differentiating early melanomas from benign naevi

A	**A**symmetry (melanoma lesion more likely to be asymmetrical)
B	**B**order irregularity (melanoma more likely to have irregular borders)
C	**C**olour (melanoma more likely to be very dark black or blue and to have variation in colour than would a benign mole, which more often is uniform in colour and light tan or brown)
D	**D**iameter (mole <6 mm in diameter usually benign)

Pathophysiology for Nurses at a Glance, First Edition. Muralitharan Nair and Ian Peate. © 2015 John Wiley & Sons, Ltd. Published 2015 by John Wiley & Sons, Ltd.
Companion website: www.ataglanceseries.com/nursing/pathophysiology

Melanocytes

Melanocytes are found in the basal layer of the epidermis the stratum basale, branching out between the keratinocytes in the suprabasal layers. Approximately 5–10% of the cells in the epidermis are melanocytes (Figure 62.1). They are found in equal numbers in black and in white skin, but the melanocytes in black skin produce more melanin. The differences in skin colour are the result of differences in the amount of melanin and the size of the melanin 'packets' that each melanocyte makes. People with dark brown or black skin are much less likely to be damaged by ultraviolet (UV) radiation than those with white skin. Non-cancerous growth of melanocytes results in moles (benign melanocytic naevi) and freckles (ephelides and lentigines). Melanin protects the skin from ultraviolet (UV) radiation, the harmful rays of the sun (Figure 62.2).

A mole is a cluster of melanocytes that appears as a pigmented spot on the skin. Moles can be either flat or raised, round or oval. They are generally benign and unchanging, they can become cancerous. The first sign of melanoma is often a change in the size, shape, or colour of an existing mole or the appearance of a new mole in adulthood.

Skin cancer

Skin cancer is the most common form of cancer in the UK. The incidence of skin cancer varies geographically; it peaks at high altitude and sunny regions. Skin cancer is more common in light skinned people than dark skinned people; however, all skin types are at risk.

Malignant melanoma

Malignant melanoma is a neoplasm of melanocytes or a neoplasm of the cells that have developed from melanocytes. Once considered uncommon, the annual incidence of malignancy has increased considerably over the past twenty years. One factor that may account for this increase in incidence is the increase in recreational activity that is taking place outdoors. Cancerous growth of melanocytes results in melanoma; most melanomas are from the skin but malignant melanomas have been described in almost every organ of the body.

Surgery is the definitive treatment for early-stage melanoma, with medical management generally reserved for adjuvant treatment of advanced melanoma.

Pathophysiology

Most skin melanomas spread out within the epidermis. If all the melanoma cells are confined to the epidermis then the lesion is a melanoma *in situ*, which can be treated by excision as it has no potential to spread. When the cancer has grown through the dermis it is known as invasive melanoma.

Four clinical types of skin melanoma exist. They are: lentigo melanoma, superficial melanoma, nodular melanoma and acral lentiginous melanoma. Nodular melanoma is the most aggressive type. It presents as a rapidly growing pigmented nodule which bleeds or ulcerates.

When the melanoma cells reach the dermis, they can spread to other tissues via the lymphatic system to the local lymph nodes, or via the bloodstream, to other organs. Metastases can occur almost anywhere and at any time after a diagnosis of melanoma. Common sites for metastases are lymph nodes, liver, lung, bone and brain. In-transit metastases are deposits from a focus of cells moving along regional lymphatic channels.

Melanomas have two growth phases, radial and vertical. During the radial growth phase, malignant cells grow in a radial fashion in the epidermis. As time passes, most melanomas progress to the vertical growth phase, in which the malignant cells invade the dermis and develop the ability to metastasize. Clinically, lesions are classified as thin if they are 1 mm or less in depth; moderate if they are 1–4 mm in depth and thick if they are greater than 4 mm in depth.

Melanoma occurs from a radiation-induced decrease in the function of the skin's immune cells – the Langerhans cells. This results in the skin being unable to identify and repair DNA damage, thereby increasing carcinogenesis.

Signs and symptoms

The melanoma may appear as a multi-coloured nodule that grows vertically or in a circular spread of pigmentation larger than 1 cm. The borders of lesions are irregular and usually asymmetrical; bleeding may occur. The melanoma may appear on sun-exposed areas or on the palms of the hands or the soles of the feet, the oral or vaginal muscosa.

A total-body skin examination is essential when evaluating a patient with an atypical naevus or a melanoma, to assess the total number of naevi present on the patient's skin. The ABCDs for differentiating early melanomas from benign naevi are in Table 62.1.

Investigations

Investigation is mainly by visual inspection and biopsy for histology, where necessary. Diagnosis should be based on a full thickness excisional biopsy. A dermatoscope can be used to examine skin lesions. Sentinel lymph node biopsy, identifying and removing the lymph node(s), immediately draining the area of the primary tumour for histological analysis, provides prognostic information and is used for pathological staging. Further investigations include chest X-ray and liver ultrasound, or CT scan of the chest, abdomen and pelvis. Blood tests include full blood count and liver function test. Only if there is indication of bone disease, should a bone scan be performed.

Staging of primary melanoma is based on the histological features of the lesion. Accurate staging is vital to determine appropriate treatment, follow-up and calculation of risk of recurrence.

Management

Primary treatment for malignant melanoma is wide local excision. Re-excision should be performed for proven melanomas if the margins are inadequate. Chemotherapy has limited benefit and response rates are limited. Dacarbazine remains the standard of care. Radiotherapy has only a limited role in the management of patients with melanoma, but it may be useful and potentially curative in some people with lentigo maligna and is sometimes used in the palliative treatment of symptomatic metastases, especially in brain and bone. For some people with advanced disease, management may focus on palliative care.

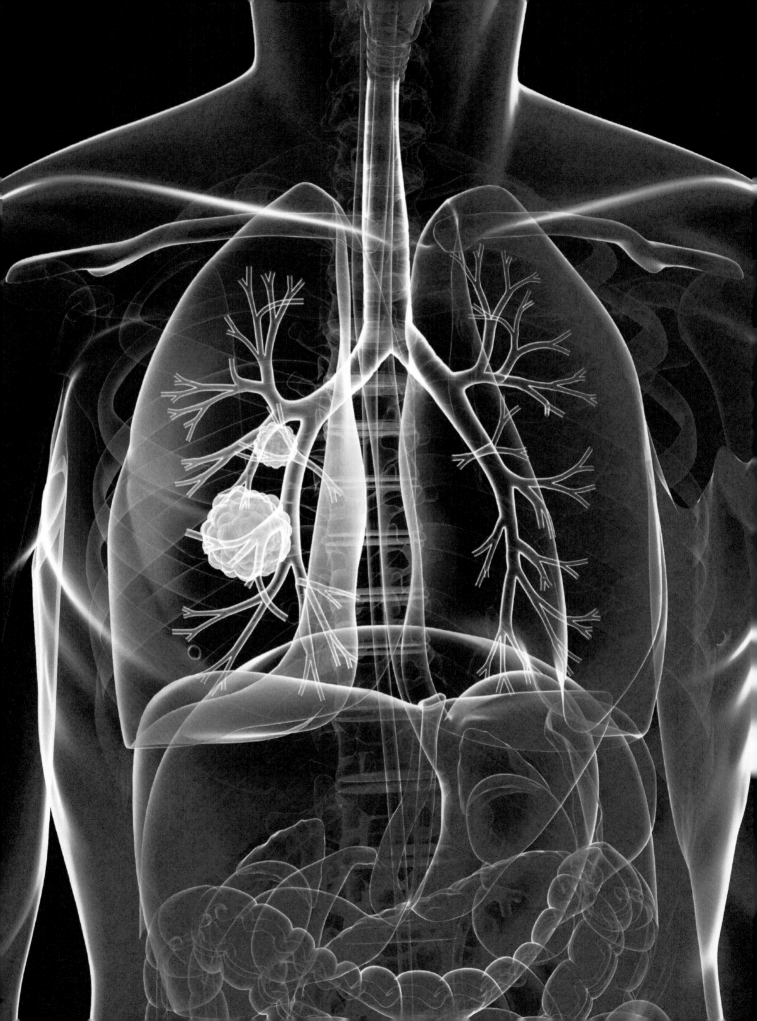

Ear, nose and throat

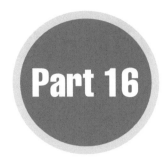

Part 16

Chapters

63 Otitis media

Figure 63.1 The ear

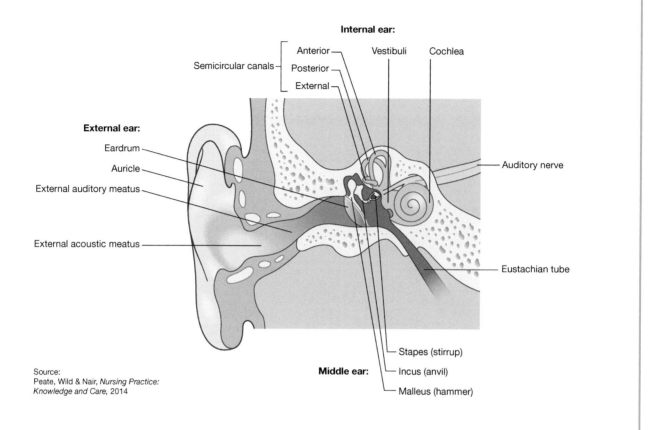

Internal ear:

External ear:

Semicircular canals
- Anterior
- Posterior
- External

Vestibuli

Cochlea

Eardrum

Auricle

External auditory meatus

External acoustic meatus

Auditory nerve

Eustachian tube

Stapes (stirrup)

Middle ear:

Incus (anvil)

Malleus (hammer)

Source:
Peate, Wild & Nair, *Nursing Practice:
Knowledge and Care*, 2014

Figure 63.2 Otitis media

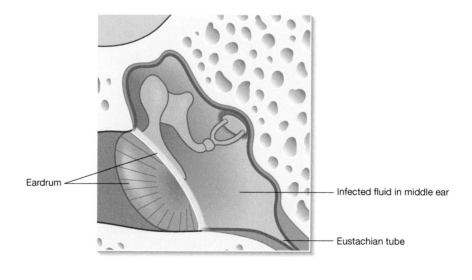

Eardrum

Infected fluid in middle ear

Eustachian tube

Otitis

Otitis refers to inflammation of the ear (Figure 63.1). Inflammation can be of the external ear – otitis externa or of the middle ear – otitis media. Otitis media is divided into two groups – acute otitis media and otitis media with effusion. Both conditions occur predominantly in childhood (but not exclusively) and can be caused by bacterial or viral infection.

Otitis media

This common condition is often seen in general practice. Most children will have a self-limiting illness; however, there will be some who will have recurrent or chronic problems and may require treatment.

As children grow, the angle between the Eustachian tube and the pharynx becomes more acute; coughing or sneezing tends to push it shut. In small children, the less acute angle enables infected material to be transmitted down the tube into the middle ear.

Pathogenesis

In the UK more than two-thirds of children experience one or more attacks of acute otitis media by the age of three and about half experience more than three episodes. The peak age of incidence is 6–24 months, the risk decreases with age. Otitis media occurs more in the winter than summer months and it is usually associated with a cold. There are a number of risk factors associated with otitis media. Boys are slightly more likely than girls to develop acute otitis media. Those children with older siblings at school or nursery are exposed to infections that may be brought home. Children who use a dummy are at increased risk; it is assumed that sucking and swallowing opens the Eustachian tube putting the middle ear at risk. Parental smoking is thought to be associated with an increase in acute and chronic otitis media.

The most important antecedent event associated with acute otitis media is obstruction of the Eustachian tube. The vast majority of acute otitis media episodes are triggered by an upper respiratory tract infection involving the nasopharynx. Usually it is a virus that is responsible for the infection. However, allergic and other inflammatory conditions involving the Eustachian tube can also result in a similar outcome. Inflammation in the nasopharynx extends to the medial end of the Eustachian tube, creating stasis and inflammation, this, in turn, alters the pressure within the middle ear. These changes may be either negative or positive, relative to ambient pressure (see Figure 63.2).

Stasis also permits pathogenic bacteria to colonize the usually sterile middle ear space through direct extension from the nasopharynx. This occurs by reflux, aspiration or active insufflation.

The most usual response is the establishment of an acute inflammatory reaction characterized by vasodilatation, exudation, leukocyte invasion, phagocytosis and local immunological responses within the middle ear cleft, which yields the clinical pattern associated with acute otitis media.

In a small number of otitis-prone children, the Eustachian tube is patulous (it lies open) or hypotonic. Children with neuromuscular disorders or abnormalities of the first or second arch are predisposed to reflux of nasopharyngeal contents into the middle ear cleft.

In order to become pathogenic in a hollow organ, for example the ear or sinus, most bacteria have to adhere to the mucosal lining. Viral infections that attack and damage mucosal linings of respiratory tracts may facilitate the ability of the bacteria to become pathogenic in the nasopharynx and Eustachian tube, as well as the middle ear cleft.

Viral infection in the nasopharynx, with subsequent inflammation of the orifice and mucosa of the Eustachian tube has long been understood as part of the pathogenesis of acute otitis media; however, the role of the virus is not fully understood. Concurrent or antecedent upper respiratory tract infections have been identified in at least 25% of all attacks of acute otitis media in children; the virus itself, however, rarely appears as the pathogen in the middle ear.

Immunological activity may play an important role in the frequency of acute otitis media and its outcome.

The immunological elements of acute otitis media are not limited to the middle ear. The nasopharynx plays an important role in the pathogenesis of acute otitis media and immunological modifications in this lymphoid tissue provide some protection from pathogens by blocking their adherence to surfaces of the mucosa.

Signs and symptoms

Where there is inflammation of the middle ear, this often occurs in association with an upper respiratory tract infection. There may be otalgia, malaise, irritability, pyrexia and vomiting. The pyrexia may be accompanied with febrile convulsions. Examination may reveal red and possibly bulging eardrums, the outer ear can sometimes glow red and there may be hearing loss. The tympanic membrane can rupture and there may be otorrhoea.

Investigations

Often no investigation is needed. Otoscopic examination may help to provide information concerning the tympanic membrane and the diagnosis of acute otitis media. Culture of discharge from an ear may be required in chronic or recurrent perforation or if there are grommets present. Audiometry should be performed if chronic hearing loss is suspected but not during the acute stage. It may be appropriate to perform a CT or MRI scan if complications are suspected.

Management

Most cases of acute otitis media resolve spontaneously and do not require treatment. Adequate analgesia and antipyretics should be prescribed in all cases, antibiotics should be avoided in mild to moderate cases and when there is diagnostic uncertainty in those aged two years and under. Antibiotic therapy should be considered for those with symptoms persisting for more than 2–3 days, children under two years with bilateral acute otitis media or bulging drum and four or more symptoms, any person with otorrhoea and those at high risk of complications, significant heart, lung, renal, liver or neuromuscular disease, immunosuppression or cystic fibrosis and young children who were born prematurely. Antibiotics are the only medications with demonstrated efficacy in the management of acute otitis media. Most antibiotics can be administered once or twice daily, improving compliance and avoiding the necessity of sending medication to school or day care centres.

64 Ménière's disease

Figure 64.1 (a) Normal membranous labyrinth and (b) dilated membranous labyrinth in Ménière's disease

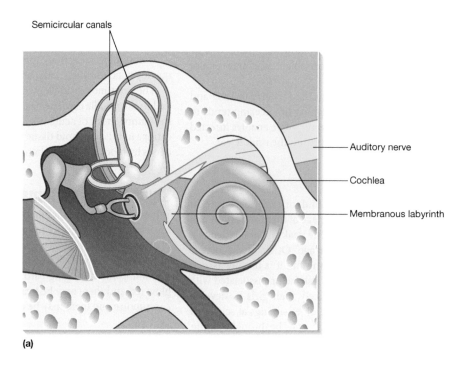

Semicircular canals

Auditory nerve

Cochlea

Membranous labyrinth

(a)

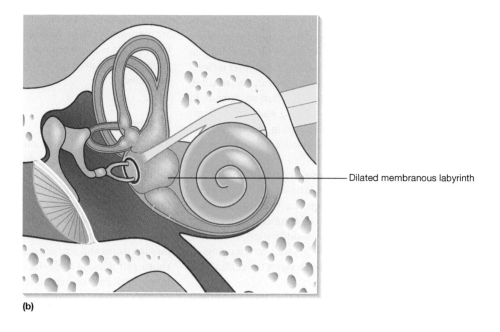

Dilated membranous labyrinth

(b)

Pathophysiology for Nurses at a Glance, First Edition. Muralitharan Nair and Ian Peate. © 2015 John Wiley & Sons, Ltd. Published 2015 by John Wiley & Sons, Ltd.
Companion website: www.ataglanceseries.com/nursing/pathophysiology

Ménière's disease (also known as idiopathic endolymphatic hydrops) is a chronic disorder of the inner ear; it is caused by a change in the fluid volume in the labyrinth. The inner ear contains the cochlea (for hearing), with the vestibular apparatus (for balance). The vestibular apparatus is a collection of tubes enclosed by the membranous labyrinth. The membranous labyrinth contains a fluid called endolymph. In Ménière's disease there is a progressive distension of the membranous labyrinth, which is called 'endolymphatic hydrops' (see Figure 64.1). This may injure the vestibular system, resulting in vertigo, or the cochlea, causing hearing loss. Endolymphatic hydrops refers to a condition of increased hydraulic pressure within the inner ear endolymphatic system.

The reported occurrence varies widely. Bilateral disease is found in 10% of patients when initially diagnosed; with disease progression, it may be found in more than 40%. Familial predisposition may be a factor, since half of patients have a significant family history. Ménière's disease can be seen at almost all ages, being noted in children as young as four years and in elderly persons older than 90 years. Onset typically begins at early to middle adulthood; peak incidence is in the 40–60-year-old age group. The condition appears to be more common in females than in males. The disease primarily affects white people.

Ménière's disease is idiopathic. If the cause of the disease is known, the disease process is no longer called Ménière's disease. However, because the origin of the problem is elevated endolymphatic pressure, it is useful to think of other causes of endolymphatic hydrops. Ménière's disease must be distinguished from these causes. Disorders that may give rise to elevated endolymphatic pressure include metabolic disturbances, hormonal imbalance, trauma and a number of various infections. Lupus and rheumatoid arthritis auto-immune diseases may cause an inflammatory response within the labyrinth. Allergy has always been linked in patients with difficult-to-treat Ménière's disease. Food triggers are also important factors in the generation of hydrops.

Pathophysiology

The exact pathophysiology of Ménière's disease is debatable. The underlying mechanism is believed to be a distortion of the membranous labyrinth, resulting from over accumulation of endolymph. The endolymph and perilymph (fluids that fill the chambers of the inner ear) are separated by thin membranes housing the neural apparatus of hearing and balance. Variations in pressure stress these nerve-rich membranes, resulting in hearing disturbance, tinnitus, vertigo, imbalance and a pressure sensation in the ear.

When hydrops occurs this is possibly due to an increase in endolymphatic pressure; in turn this causes a break in the membrane that separates the perilymph from the endolymph. The sudden change in the rate of vestibular nerve firing creates an acute vestibular imbalance. The actual distention caused by increased endolymphatic pressure also leads to a mechanical disturbance of the auditory and otolithic organs. Irritation of the utricle and saccule may produce non-rotational vestibular symptoms.

This physical distention also results in mechanical disturbance of the organ of Corti. Distortion of the basilar membrane and the inner and outer hair cells can cause hearing loss and/or tinnitus.

Signs and symptoms

The key symptoms are vertigo and tinnitus, along with fluctuating hearing loss and a sensation of aural pressure. The key feature of the disease is its fluctuating and episodic pattern of symptoms: acute attacks can last from minutes to hours, frequently 2–3 hours. Acute episodes may occur in clusters of 6–11 per year. Remission of symptoms may last several months. Initially the majority of patients develop unilateral symptoms. Bilateral symptoms can develop, but many years later.

Other symptoms include 'drop attacks', whereby the person experiences sudden unexplained falls without loss of consciousness or related vertigo. Imbalance is sometimes reported, tending to occur once the spinning sensation has diminished.

Three stages of the disease are described (not all patients go through all these).

Early-stage: predominantly vertigo attacks, which are sudden and unpredictable, hearing worsens and tinnitus increases.

Middle-stage: continuing episodes of vertigo; there may be giddiness before and after attacks. Sensorineural hearing loss develops. Tinnitus also progresses.

Late-stage: hearing loss increases. Vertigo lessens; balance may be difficult. Tinnitus persists.

Investigations

In order to make a firm diagnosis, the following symptoms should be present: vertigo, tinnitus and hearing loss.

With Ménière's there are no diagnostic signs. Examination of other systems is advisable in order to consider causes of similar symptoms. It must be remembered that many other conditions can present with vertigo, tinnitus or deafness. Other ear, nose and throat causes could include acoustic neuroma in people with unilateral deafness, tinnitus and/or facial nerve palsy, otitis media, impacted cerumen and the use of ototoxic drugs. The clinician must be aware of the possibility of intracranial pathology.

Investigations include a range of blood tests to exclude systemic illness, for example full blood count, thyroid function, syphilis screen, fasting glucose, renal function, lipids. Audiometry is recommended to diagnose Ménière's disease if sensorineural hearing loss is found. Diagnosis can be aided by video nystagmography or electronystagmographic testing with bithermal caloric evaluation, electrocochleography and brainstem auditory evoked potentials. If unilateral, an MRI brain scan is advised to exclude other causes of unilateral vertigo and hearing loss, for example acoustic neuroma. This should include views of the internal auditory canal, with and without contrast medium.

Management

The aim of treatment is to alleviate acute attacks, reduce severity and frequency of attacks, enhance hearing and reduce the impact of tinnitus. Vertigo and nausea can be alleviated by prochloperazine cinnarizine or cyclizine; these can be given buccally or intramuscularly if vomiting is occuring. Intramuscular steroid injection followed by a reduced dose of oral steroids has also been recommended. Low-salt diet and avoiding caffeine, chocolate, alcohol and tobacco are advised. Surgical treatment is a possibility but there are side effects that the person needs to be informed about. Drivers of any type of vehicle are required to send a form to the Driver and Vehicle Licensing Agency if they have vertigo, regardless of the cause.

65 Pharyngitis

Figure 65.1 Normal and infected throat

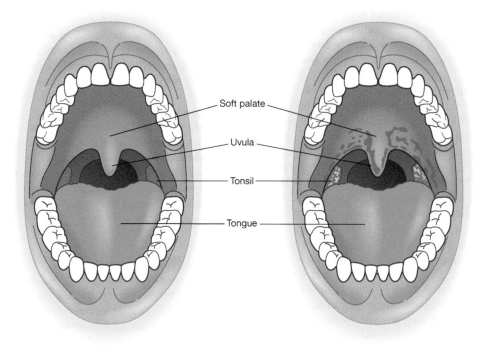

Soft palate

Uvula

Tonsil

Tongue

Normal

Pharyngitis

Figure 65.2 Taking a throat swab

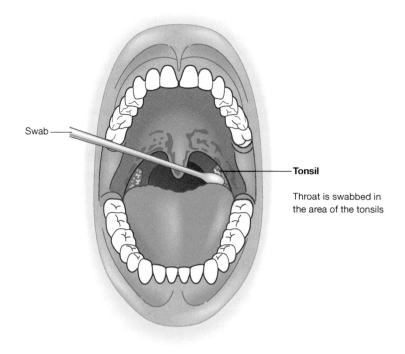

Swab

Tonsil

Throat is swabbed in
the area of the tonsils

Pathophysiology for Nurses at a Glance, First Edition. Muralitharan Nair and Ian Peate. © 2015 John Wiley & Sons, Ltd. Published 2015 by John Wiley & Sons, Ltd.
Companion website: www.ataglanceseries.com/nursing/pathophysiology

Pharyngitis

Pharyngitis is an infection or irritation of the pharynx and/or tonsils (see Figure 65.1). The cause is usually infectious; the majority of cases are viral in origin. For the most part these cases are non-threatening and self-limiting. The bacterial causes of pharyngitis are also self-limiting; however, they can cause concern because of suppurative and non-suppurative complications. Other causes of pharyngitis can include allergy, trauma, toxins and neoplasia.

The most common bacterial agent causing pharyngitis in both adults and children is group A beta-haemolytic streptococcus infection. The most common viruses are rhinovirus and adenovirus.

It is difficult to estimate the incidence of pharyngitis. It is likely to be under-reported as a result of its self-limiting nature and the person may never consult a clinician. Pharyngitis occurs with much greater frequency in the child population. The peak incidence of bacterial and viral pharyngitis occurs in the school-aged child aged 4–7 years. Pharyngitis is rare in children younger than three years. Mortality from pharyngitis is rare, but may result from one of its complications, most notably airway obstruction. Other sequelae of streptococcal pharyngitis include acute glomerulonephritis, peritonsillar abscess and toxic shock syndrome.

Pathophysiology

In infectious pharyngitis, bacteria or viruses may directly invade the mucosa of the pharynx, which causes a local inflammatory response. Viruses such as rhinovirus and coronavirus can cause irritation of pharyngeal mucosa that is secondary to nasal secretions.

Streptococcal infections are characterized by local invasion with the release of extracellular toxins and proteases. As well as this, M protein fragments (the virulent factor of the bacterium) of certain serotypes of group A beta-haemolytic streptococcus are similar to myocardial sarcolemma antigens and these are linked to rheumatic fever and subsequent heart valve damage. The prevalence rates of these serotypes of group A beta-haemolytic streptococcus have been becoming rarer over the years.

Signs and symptoms

The causes of viral and bacterial pharyngitis are similar; differentiation of the cause is difficult when this is based on history and physical examination alone. The signs and symptoms by themselves cannot be used to rule out or diagnose group A beta-haemolytic streptococcus pharyngitis. These are the classic presentations:

- Most common in children aged 4–7 years.
- Sudden onset is a feature consistent with pharyngitis.
- Pharyngitis following several days of coughing or rhinorrhoea is more consistent with a viral aetiology.
- The person has been in contact with others diagnosed with group A beta-haemolytic streptococcus or rheumatic fever presenting with symptoms consistent with group A beta-haemolytic streptococcus.
- Headache is a feature.
- Cough is not usually associated with pharyngitis infection.
- There may be vomiting

- A recent history of orogenital contact suggests the possibility of gonococcal pharyngitis.
- A history of rheumatic fever is important when considering treatment.
- Pyrexia.
- Anterior cervical lymphadenopathy.
- Tonsillar exudates.

The symptom of soreness on swallowing may be accompanied by fever and symptoms of upper respiratory tract infection, such as headache, malaise, rhinitis and cough. Hoarseness may be present if there is laryngeal involvement. The practitioner should ask about:

- Duration and severity of symptoms
- Any self-medication/over-the-counter treatment
- History of any comorbidities, previous risk factors, relevant past history
- Presence of trismus
- Feeling systemically unwell
- Dysphagia
- Stridor
- Rash

Investigations

Investigations in a primary care setting is not usually necessary. However, if symptoms and/or signs are prolonged, severe or atypical, then investigation should be considered.

Throat swab may be helpful if bacterial infection is suspected or there is exudation or excessive erythema (see Figure 65.2). A full blood count and glandular fever screening test are required (these may help if glandular fever is suspected). Antistreptolysin O (ASO) titres may be of value in excluding recent streptococcal infection in those who are systemically unwell or have prolonged symptoms. A gonococcal culture should be performed as indicated by history.

Examination of the throat using a tongue depressor must never be attempted in those with stridor, as there may be epiglottitis and examination could provoke laryngeal spasm. Examination may reveal redness of the pharynx and tonsils, enlargement of the tonsils, presence of exudate and enlarged tender cervical lymph glands.

Management

Efforts should be made to make an accurate diagnosis before considering treatment, as pharyngitis is a symptom of an underlying condition. National recommendations concerning assessment of all patients presenting with sore throat are available. Sore throat is often a self-limiting condition with natural resolution in one week. It should be suggested to the person that they rest and avoid social contact to attempt to prevent transmission.

Antipyretic analgesics such as paracetamol and ibuprofen are of value. Antibiotics may be prescribed, there are three options:

1 No antibiotics
2 Delayed antibiotics
3 Immediate prescription of antibiotics

It may be necessary to administer steroids if there are any signs of airway compromise, as well as to provide symptomatic relief.

66 Rhinosinusitis

Figure 66.1 The nasal cavity

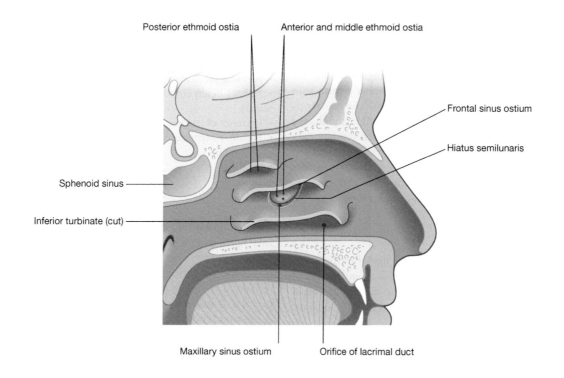

Posterior ethmoid ostia

Anterior and middle ethmoid ostia

Frontal sinus ostium

Hiatus semilunaris

Sphenoid sinus

Inferior turbinate (cut)

Maxillary sinus ostium

Orifice of lacrimal duct

Figure 66.2 Symptoms of rhinosinusitis

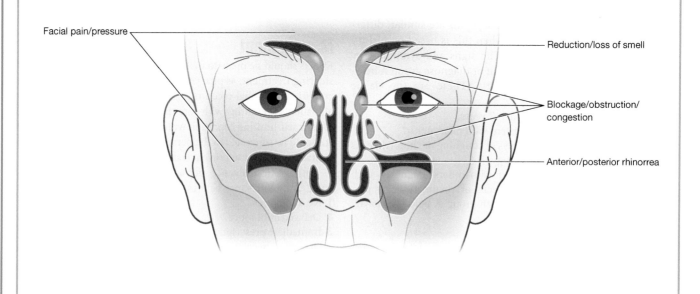

Facial pain/pressure

Reduction/loss of smell

Blockage/obstruction/ congestion

Anterior/posterior rhinorrea

Pathophysiology for Nurses at a Glance, First Edition. Muralitharan Nair and Ian Peate. © 2015 John Wiley & Sons, Ltd. Published 2015 by John Wiley & Sons, Ltd.
Companion website: www.ataglanceseries.com/nursing/pathophysiology

Rhinosinusitis

The nasal cavity is illustrated in Figure 66.1. Sinusitis is characterized by inflammation of the lining of the paranasal sinuses. The preferred term for the condition is rhinosinustits, because the nasal mucosa is simultaneously involved and because sinusitis seldom occurs without concurrent rhinitis. The paranasal sinuses refer to the frontal, maxillary, sphenoidal and ethmoidal sinuses. They develop as diverticula from the nasal mucosa and are elementary or absent at birth, only expanding rapidly during the eruption of permanent teeth and again at puberty.

As a result of referred pain the paranasal sinuses may cause diagnostic problems: innervation of the maxilliary sinus is by the infraorbital nerve and anterior, middle and posterior superior alveolar nerves. As a result of this the pathology here can be experienced as upper jaw pain, toothache or pain in the skin of the cheek.

Rhinosinusitis is a very common condition that affects around 15% of the population in Western countries and is more prevalent in winter than in summer.

An average child is likely to have 6–8 upper respiratory tract infections per year, which may be complicated by the development of acute bacterial sinusitis. Women have more occurrences of infective sinusitis than men; this may be because they tend to have closer contact with young children.

Pathophysiology

Usually the sinuses are sterile. Secretions produced in the sinuses under ciliary action flow through the ostia, draining into the nasal cavity. The flow of sinus secretions in healthy people is always unidirectional, towards the ostia; this stops contamination of the sinuses. In the majority of people, the maxillary sinus has a single ostium acting as the solitary outflow tract for drainage. In a nondependent position the thin channel rests high on the medial wall of the sinus cavity. More than likely, the oedema of the mucosa at these openings becomes congested by some means, for example allergy, viruses, chemical irritation causing obstruction of the outflow tract, stasis of secretions with negative pressure, leading to infection by bacteria.

Mucus that has become infected, leads to sinusitis. Another mechanism suggests that as the sinuses are continuous with the nasal cavity, colonized bacteria in the nasopharynx may contaminate the sterile sinuses. These bacteria are usually removed by mucociliary clearance; thus, if mucociliary clearance changes, bacteria may be inoculated and infection may occur, leading to sinusitis.

Rhinosinusitis is divided into categories in relation to how long the illness lasts (temporal classification).

Acute: lasting 7–30 days, sub-acute lasts 4–12 weeks.

Recurring: where there are more than three significant acute episodes in a year lasting for ten days or more with no intervening symptoms.

Chronic: symptoms persist for longer than 90 days (can be caused by irreversible changes in the mucosal lining of the sinuses), with or without acute exacerbations.

Viral disease lasts less than ten days, whereas worsening symptoms after five days or symptoms extending beyond ten days suggest bacterial infection.

Signs and symptoms

There is no specific clinical symptom or sign that is sensitive or specific for acute sinusitis; therefore the overall clinical impression is used to guide management.

Acute sinusitis usually follows an upper respiratory tract infection and is diagnosed by the presence of obstruction/congestion, **or** anterior/posterior nasal drip **with** facial pain (or pressure) and/or reduction of, or loss of, the sense of smell,

Nasal discharge – a thick, purulent, green coloured discharge is more likely to indicate bacterial involvement. Nasal blockage or congestion – often bilateral is caused by rhinitis. Facial pain is described as pressure and localized over the infected sinus, or it can affect teeth, the upper jaw, or other areas (such as eye, side of face, forehead). Pain in the absence of other symptoms is unlikely to be sinusitis. See Figure 66.2.

Investigations

Investigations are not necessary to diagnose acute sinusitis, this is a controversial area. Examination is of limited value but may reveal the presence of purulent discharge, swelling of the nasal mucosa and tenderness over the sinuses. However, anterior rhinoscopic examination, with or without a topical decongestant, is important in assessing the status of the nasal mucosa and the presence and colour of nasal discharge. Predisposing anatomical variations can also be noted during anterior rhinoscopy. Endoscopic examination can demonstrate the origin of the purulent discharge and can offer information about the nature of ostiomeatal obstruction.

Management
Acute sinusitis

Diagnosis is made on the history and the presenting signs and symptoms. The person should be reassured that this is generally a viral infection similar to a cold but which takes a little longer to resolve. Measures to relieve symptoms include paracetamol/ibuprofen for pain/fever, intranasal decongestant for a maximum of a week and nasal irrigation with warm saline solution. Warm face packs, can offer localized pain relief. Antibiotics are given for severe or prolonged infections (longer than five days). If the person's condition is deteriorating, management may involve microbiological investigation, intravenous antibiotics, sinus puncture and irrigation sinus surgery to restore sinus ventilation and mucociliary function.

Chronic sinusitis

Chronic sinusitis cases can be divided into three principal types: those without polyps, those with polyps and those associated with fungal infection. The condition is less common than acute sinusitis. Symptoms are similar to those of acute sinusitis but not as florid. There may be a dull ache on palpation and nasal mucosal inflammation may be noted.

The diagnostic criteria are as for acute sinusitis with symptoms lasting for more than 12 weeks. Investigations are not usually needed. Management in the first instance is medical, regardless of the presence of polyps. Administration of beclometasone 50 micrograms nasal spray treatment is given. As with acute sinusitis, management is aimed at restoring sinus ventilation.

67 Epistaxis

Figure 67.1 Cross section of the nasal cavity and vasculature

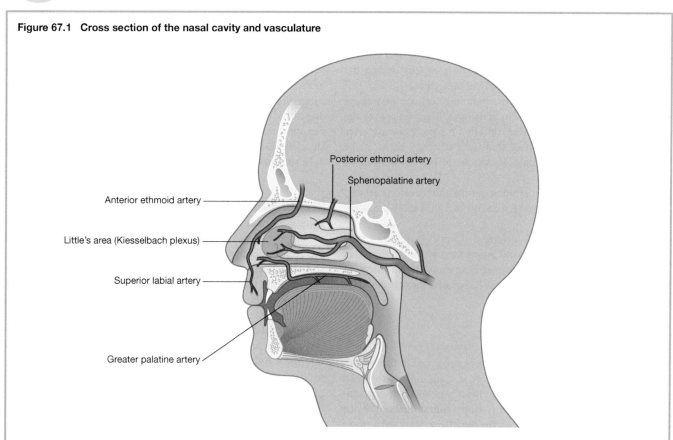

Anterior ethmoid artery

Little's area (Kiesselbach plexus)

Superior labial artery

Greater palatine artery

Posterior ethmoid artery

Sphenopalatine artery

Pathophysiology for Nurses at a Glance, First Edition. Muralitharan Nair and Ian Peate. © 2015 John Wiley & Sons, Ltd. Published 2015 by John Wiley & Sons, Ltd.
Companion website: www.ataglanceseries.com/nursing/pathophysiology

Epistaxis

Epistaxes (nose bleeds) are usually self-limiting and harmless, often the cause of damage to the blood vessels is not identified. It is rare that they are life threatening. However, they can cause significant concern, particularly for the parents of small children. Most epistaxes originate from Little's area on the anterior nasal septum, which contains the Kiesselbach plexus of vessels (see Figure 67.1). Rarely, epistaxis originates from branches of the sphenopalatine artery in the posterior nasal cavity.

Over half of the population has experienced an episode of epistaxis. The true prevalence of epistaxis is not known, as most episodes are self-limited and as such they are not reported. The incidence of epistaxis changes with age. Peaks in incidence occur in children younger than ten years of age and in adults older than 45 years of age. It is unusual for children younger than two years of age to have an epistaxis; when they do it may be associated with injury or serious illness. In older people posterior epistaxis is more common compared with younger people.

Pathophysiology

There are a number of causes of epistaxis and they can be divided into local causes such as: trauma; mucosal irritation; septal abnormality; inflammatory diseases; tumours; systemic causes, for example blood dyscrasias, arteriosclerosis, hereditary haemorrhagic telangiectasia; as well as idiopathic causes. The most common cause is local trauma, followed by facial trauma, foreign bodies, nasal or sinus infections and sustained inhalation of dry air. Self-induced trauma (nasal picking) can result in anterior septal mucosal ulceration and bleeding. This is often the case in young children. Nasal foreign bodies causing local trauma such as nasogastric and nasotracheal tubes may also be responsible for rare cases of epistaxis. Acute facial and nasal trauma frequently leads to epistaxis. If the bleeding is the result of minor mucosal laceration, usually this is limited. In extensive facial trauma this can result in severe bleeding requiring nasal packing. Nasal surgery has the potential to cause epistaxis; this may range from minor, as a result of mucosal laceration, to severe, due to transection of a major vessel. Mucosal irritation can be the result of low humidity. In dry climates and during cold weather epistaxis is more prevalent as a result of the dehumidification of the nasal mucosa by home heating systems. The administration of topical nasal drugs such as antihistamines and corticosteroids can lead to mucosal irritation, causing mild epistaxis. Medications such as non-steroidal anti-inflammatory drugs (NSAIDs) are also frequently involved. Septal deviations and spurs have the potential to disrupt the normal nasal airflow, this can lead to dryness and epistaxis. The bleeding sites are often situated anterior to the spurs in most people. The edges of septal perforations often harbour crusting and are common sources of epistaxis. Bacterial, viral and allergic rhinosinusitis results in mucosal inflammation and can lead to epistaxis. When bleeding occurs in these cases it is usually minor, often manifesting as blood-streaked nasal discharge. Granulomatosis diseases such as sarcoidosis, Wegener granulomatosis, tuberculosis, syphilis and rhinoscleroma can sometimes lead to crusting and friable mucosa; this may be a cause of recurring epistaxis.

Benign and malignant tumours can come across as epistaxis. Those people affected can also present with signs and symptoms of nasal obstruction and rhinosinusitis that is usually unilateral.

Blood dyscrasias, including congenital coagulopathies, should be considered in those with a positive family history, easy bruising, or prolonged bleeding from minor trauma or surgery. Examples of congenital bleeding disorders are haemophilia and von Willebrand disease.

Acquired coagulopathies can be due to the diseases or to their treatments. The more common acquired coagulopathies are thrombocytopaenia and liver disease. Oral anticoagulants predispose to epistaxis. Cocaine use, usually taken by inhalation, has a very strong vasoconstrictive effect that can lead to complete obliteration of the nasal septum and cause epistaxis

Arteriosclerotic vascular disease is believed to be a reason for the higher prevalence of epistaxis in older people. The Kiesselbach plexus, a part of the trigeminovascular system, has been implicated in the pathogenesis of migraine. The relationship between hypertension and epistaxis is often misunderstood. Those with epistaxis often present with hypertension, and epistaxis is more prevalent in those with hypertension, this may be due to vascular fragility as a result of long-standing disease. It is rare for hypertension to be a direct cause of epistaxis. Epistaxis and the associated anxiety this brings can cause an acute elevation of blood pressure.

In some case the cause of epistaxis is not always readily identifiable (idiopathic).

Signs and symptoms

Establish if blood is running out of the nose and one nostril (usually anterior) or if blood is running into the throat or from both nostrils (usually posterior). Ask about trauma (including nose picking). Note family or past history of clotting disorders or hypertension. Determine whether there has been previous nasal surgery. Consider medication, especially anticoagulants. Ask about any facial pain or otalgia.

Investigations

Laboratory studies are not usually needed for first-time nosebleeds or infrequent recurrences with a good history of nose picking or trauma to the nose. However, they are required if major bleeding is present or if a coagulopathy is suspected.

Management

When medical attention is needed for epistaxis, it is usually because the problem is either recurrent or severe. Treatment depends on the clinical picture. Bleeding responds to cauterization, nasal packing, or both. For those who have recurrent or severe bleeding for which medical therapy has failed, a number of surgical options are available. After surgery or embolization, patients should be closely observed for any complications or signs of rebleeding. Adequate pain control is needed for people with nasal packing, especially in those with posterior packing. Oral and topical antibiotics are given to prevent rhinosinusitis and possibly toxic shock syndrome. Avoid aspirin and other non-steroidal anti-inflammatory drugs. Medications to control underlying medical problems (such as hypertension, vitamin K deficiency) may be given in consultation with other specialists.

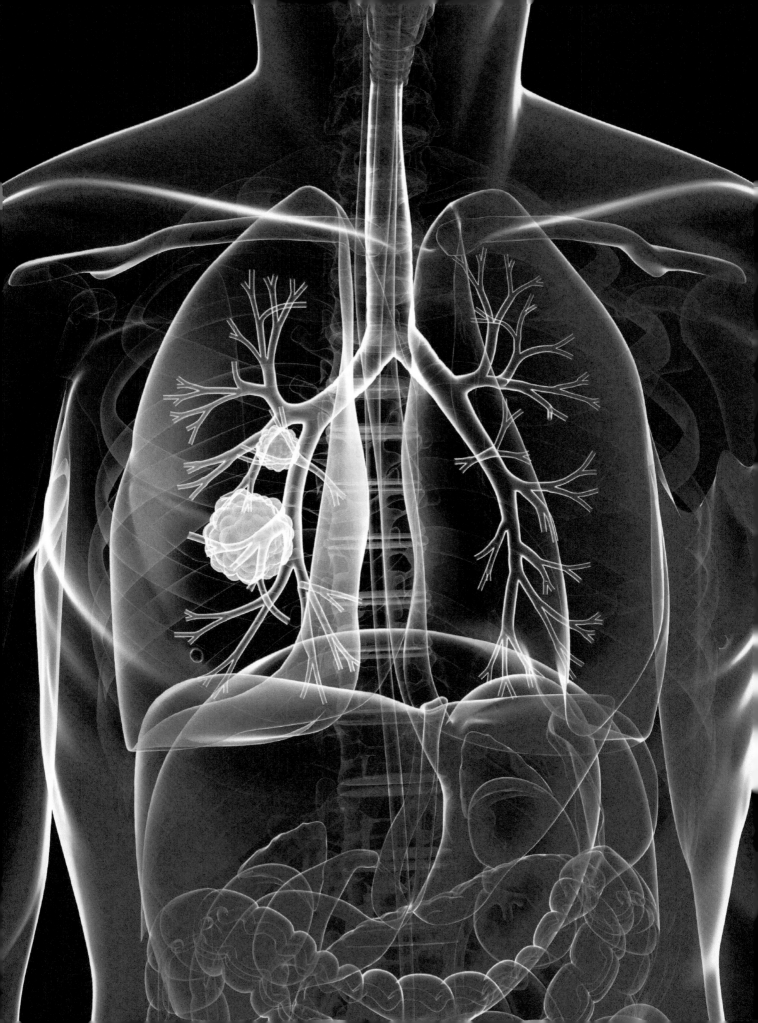

Vision

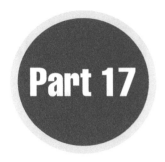

Part 17

Chapters

68 Cataracts

Figure 68.1 The eye

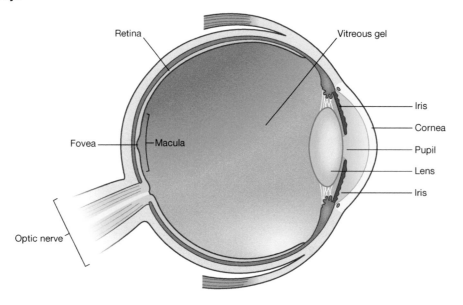

Retina — Vitreous gel — Iris — Cornea — Pupil — Lens — Iris — Fovea — Macula — Optic nerve

Figure 68.2 Normal lens (a) and lens affected by cataract (b)

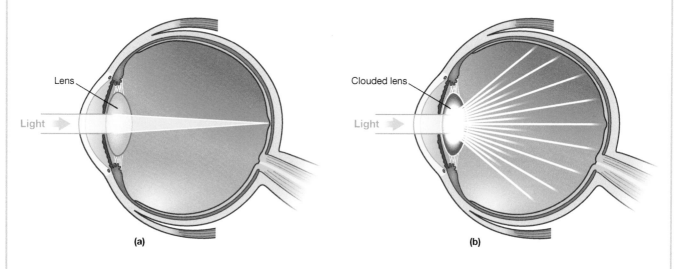

Lens

Light

(a)

Clouded lens

Light

(b)

Figure 68.3 Phacoemulsification

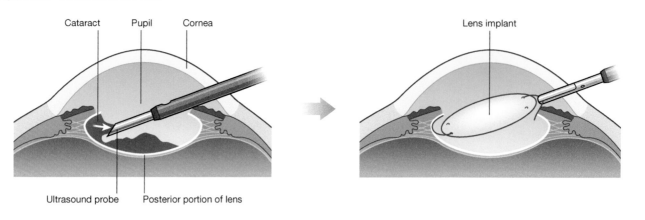

Cataract — Pupil — Cornea — Lens implant — Ultrasound probe — Posterior portion of lens

Cataract is an age-related, vision-impairing disease characterized by slow, progressive thickening of the lens of the eye. Globally it is one of the leading causes of blindness. Cataracts are lens opacities that can range in severity from unnoticed dots to total fogging. Whilst the main cause is deterioration of a lens with age, congenital cataracts can also occur.

Cataract

Age-related cataract is reversible. Over time a cataract can get worse, gradually making vision mistier. Early detection, close monitoring and timely surgical intervention must be undertaken in the management of cataracts.

When light passes through the front of the eye it is focused by the cornea and then the lens onto the retina (see Figure 68.1). The lens is normally clear, enabling that light to pass directly through to focus on the retina (the lens is clear due to the way the cells in the lens are arranged). The lens focuses light onto the retina, which converts the light into electrical signals. A network of nerves delivers these signals from the different parts of the retina to the optic nerve and then onto the brain. The brain interprets these signals to 'see' the world around us.

Cataracts result from changes in the way the cells of the lens are arranged and their water content, this results in the lens becoming cloudy as opposed to clear (see Figure 68.2). When this occurs, light cannot pass directly through the lens and problems with vision may occur. A cataract is not a tumour or a sheet growing over the eye, it is the lens becoming misty.

Pathophysiology

Apart from age, the following risk factors for cataract include female gender, diabetes mellitus, use of steroids, eye trauma, UV exposure, uveitis, poor nutrition and socioeconomic status, smoking and use of alcohol.

The pathophysiology concerning cataracts is complex and is not fully understood. The pathogenesis is multifactorial, involving complex interactions between a number of physiological processes. As the lens ages, its weight and thickness increases, whilst its ability to accommodate decreases. As new cortical layers are added in a concentric manner, the central nucleus is compressed and becomes hardened as a result of nuclear sclerosis.

A number of mechanisms contribute to the progressive loss of transparency of the lens. The epithelium of the lens is thought to experience age-related changes, especially a decrease in lens epithelial cell density and an aberrant differentiation of lens fibre cells. Although the epithelium of the lens with cataract experiences a low rate of apoptotic death, which is unlikely to result in a significant decrease in cell density, the accumulation of small-scale epithelial losses may subsequently result in a modification of lens fibre formation and homeostasis. This will lead to loss of lens transparency. As the lens ages, there is a reduction in the rate at which water can enter the cells of the lens nucleus via the epithelium and cortex, with an ensuing reduction in the rate of transport of water, nutrients and antioxidants.

Three types of age-related cataracts occur:
1 Nuclear sclerosis, this cataract is formed by new layers of fibre (added with ageing) compressing the nucleus of the lens.
2 Cortical, new fibres are added to the outside of the lens, which age and produce cortical spokes. These may not cause symptoms unless on the visual axis, or the entire cortex is affected when it is 'mature'.
3 Posterior subcapsular opacities in the central posterior cortex. This can happen in younger people and can cause glare with or without deterioration in near vision.

Signs and symptoms

There may be one or both eyes affected. Co-existing eye conditions such as glaucoma, age-related macular degeneration, diabetic retinopathy and amblyopia are frequently present in those who require cataract surgery.

Typical symptoms are slow painless loss of vision, problems with reading, failing to recognize faces, problems watching TV and diplopia in one eye. Opacities can be seen as defects in the red reflex when the ophthalmoscope is held 60 cm from the eye; the pupil should be dilated to see this clearly. As a bright light is shone onto the eye the lens can appear brown or white.

Investigations

After a thorough history is taken, careful physical examination must be performed. The eye is checked for abnormalities that may point out systemic illnesses that affect the eye and the development of cataract. Diagnosis is made after a thorough history and physical examination have been performed.

Management

Failure to treat a developing cataract surgically can lead to damaging consequences, such as lens swelling and intumescence, secondary glaucoma or even, eventually, blindness.

There is no proven medical treatment that currently exists to postpone, avoid, or reverse the development of cataracts. Surgical removal of the cataract is the only effective treatment available to restore or maintain vision. Most cataract surgery in the UK is performed on older people; the majority of these people are over 60 years of age.

The most widely used surgical intervention is phacoemulsification, which is the safest and most effective technique (see Figure 68.3). There is no absolute threshold of visual acuity at which surgery is required. The impact of the cataract on the patient's quality of life is a deciding factor. In phacoemulsification an incision approximately 3 mm in diameter is made in the sclera, a round hole approximately 5 mm diameter is made in the lens capsule. Liquification of the hard lens nucleus is by the use of an ultrasonic probe inserted through the hole to extract the lens. Soft lens fibres are removed. The replacement lens is placed folded into the empty capsular bag and it unfolds. The incision will heal without sutures.

The procedure is performed on a day-case basis, using locally injected anaesthetic or anaesthetic eye drops can also be used. Topical antibiotics and steroids are required postoperatively and the person is advised to avoid of strenuous activity.

69 Glaucoma

Figure 69.1 Glaucoma

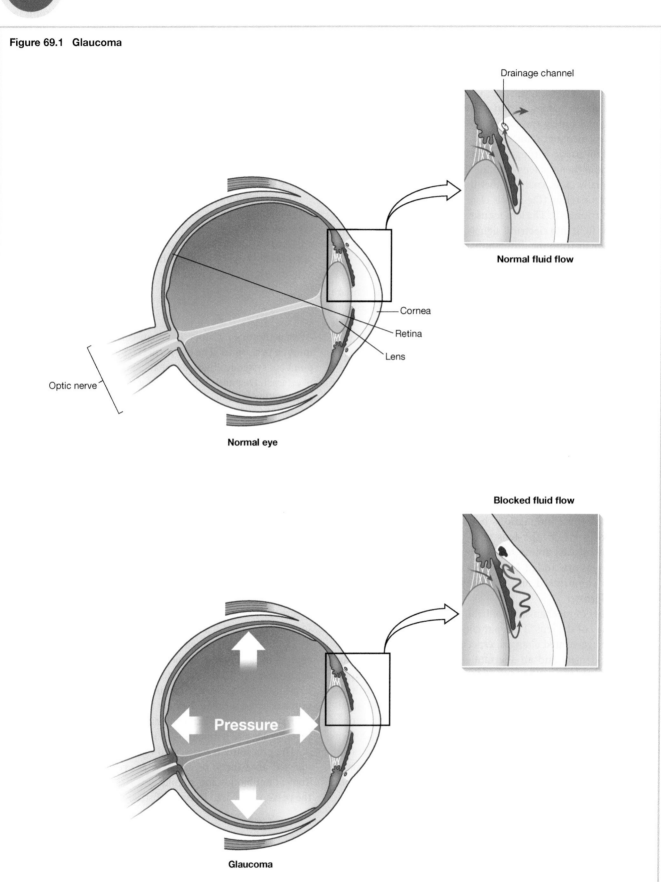

Drainage channel

Normal fluid flow

Cornea
Retina
Lens

Optic nerve

Normal eye

Blocked fluid flow

Pressure

Glaucoma

Pathophysiology for Nurses at a Glance, First Edition. Muralitharan Nair and Ian Peate. © 2015 John Wiley & Sons, Ltd. Published 2015 by John Wiley & Sons, Ltd.
Companion website: www.ataglanceseries.com/nursing/pathophysiology

Glaucoma is a condition of the eye usually caused by an abnormal increase in intra-ocular pressure, greater than 20 mm/Hg. The high pressures can sometimes reach 70–80 mm/Hg, which causes compression on the optic nerve as it leaves the eyeball.

Glaucoma is seen as a disruption of the structural or functional integrity of the optic nerve that leads to characteristic atrophic changes in the optic nerve; over time this can also lead to specific visual field defects. This disruption can usually be arrested or reduced by adequate lowering of intra-ocular pressure.

Glaucoma refers to the family of conditions characterized by optic neuropathy. The generic term glaucoma should only be used when referring to the whole group of glaucomatous disorders; there are multiple subsets of glaucomatous disease. If the specific diagnosis is known, a more precise term should be used to describe the glaucoma.

Glaucoma is classified depending on whether it is congenital or acquired. It is further subdivided into open or closed angle, depending on how the aqueous outflow is impaired. Primary or secondary types are recognized, depending on the presence of underlying related factors.

Glaucoma
Pathophysiology

In glaucoma the main problem is a disease of the optic nerve, the pathophysiology underpinning this is not fully understood. Neuropathy is associated with a raised intra-ocular pressure for most types of glaucoma. This leads to the suggestion of retinal ganglion apoptosis, the rate of which is influenced by the intra-ocular pressure itself, as it mechanically increases pressure on the head of the optic nerve and compromises the local microvasculature. Clinically, this is reflected in a gradual loss of peripheral visual field. See Figure 69.1.

Worldwide, 12.5 million people are blind from glaucoma. It accounts for 10% of registrations of blindness in the UK. Primary open angle glaucoma occurs in about 2% of people over 40 and 10% of those over 75. In England, annually there are over a million glaucoma-related hospital outpatient visits.

There are several forms of glaucoma: the two most common forms are primary open-angle glaucoma and angle-closure glaucoma.

Primary open-angle glaucoma
Signs and symptoms

Open-angle glaucoma is often called 'the sneak thief of sight' as it has no symptoms until substantial loss of sight has occurred. Usually there are no early warning signs or symptoms. It develops slowly and sometimes without noticeable sight loss for a number of years. Most people with open-angle glaucoma are well and at first do not notice a change in their vision; visual acuity is maintained until late in the disease. By the time the person becomes aware of vision loss, the disease is fairly advanced. Loss of vision from glaucoma is not reversible with treatment. Suspicion arises during the course of a routine optician check, where abnormal discs, intra-ocular pressure or visual fields may be noted. The risks for glaucoma include age, family history, Afro-Caribbean descent and if there is diabetes mellitus or a history of cardiovascular disease.

Investigations

A detailed history is taken and the eye is examined thoroughly for evidence of glaucoma, comorbidity or an alternative diagnosis to the apparent findings. Glaucoma assessment includes gonioscopy, corneal thickness assessment, tonometry and optic disc examination. Visual fields are assessed.

Management

There is much variation in management of this condition. National guidelines are available. Treatment may not necessarily be commenced immediately. The potential for variation of findings from one assessment to the next means that the patient should be assessed on several occasions unless the findings are unmistakable; the diagnosis is significant and treatment is lifelong. In those patients where the disease is obvious and advanced, treatment should commence quickly.

Medical therapy is the first-line treatment and for many patients the only treatment. Treatment may be to one or both eyes. Prostaglandin analogues have been favoured above beta blockers. Carbonic anhydrase inhibitors may be prescribed. Sympathomimetic and miotics can be used. Laser and surgical treatments should be considered after unsuccessful trials with two different pharmacological treatments.

Angle-closure glaucoma
Signs and symptoms

The person with acute-closure glaucoma is generally unwell, complaining of severe pain with a progressively rapid onset; it may be confined to the eye but often spreads around the orbit with an associated frontal or generalized headache. There may be blurred vision, progressing quickly to visual loss; the person may see coloured haloes around lights. The person may describe subacute attacks where there is a history of transient blurring of vision and haloes around light. Systemic malaise in the form of nausea and vomiting are common and may be the main presenting feature.

Investigations

Diagnosis is made on history and examination. Examination of the eye shows a red eye with a hazy cornea and a non-reactive (or minimally reactive) mid-dilated pupil. The globe is hard on palpation and the intra-ocular pressure will be raised.

The acute attack is often unilateral; however, predisposing factors are bilateral and long-term management will be to both eyes.

Management

The paramount concern (day or night) is to reduce the intra-ocular pressure and save the sight. Topical agents include beta blockers, steroids, apraclonidine, pilocarpine (for those with a natural lens) after starting treatment, or phenylephrine in those with a history of a cataract extraction in the past. Acetazolamide is given intravenously. If there is no response, systemic hyperosmotics, such as glycerol are given orally or mannitol 20% solution IV 1–1.5 gm/kg may be added. Systemic analgesia and antiemetics should be offered.

Subsequent treatment is aimed at specific mechanism of closure through surgical intervention.

70 Age-related macular degeneration

Figure 70.1   The eye showing the position of the macula

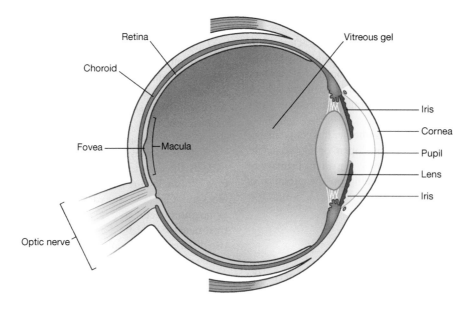

Figure 70.2   Normal macula and degenerated

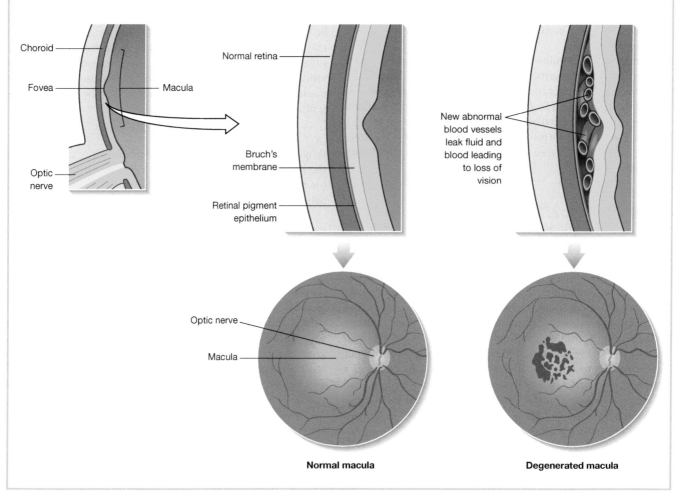

Pathophysiology for Nurses at a Glance, First Edition. Muralitharan Nair and Ian Peate. © 2015 John Wiley & Sons, Ltd. Published 2015 by John Wiley & Sons, Ltd.
Companion website: www.ataglanceseries.com/nursing/pathophysiology

ARMD is also known as age-related macular degeneration.

The macula

Age-related macular degeneration affects the macula area of the retina. This is a very small area of the retina that plays a central role in seeing detail, colour and things immediately in front of the person (see Figure 70.1). When the light enters the eye it is focused onto the retina at the back of the eye. The retina includes a number of layers; however, the most important for vision is a layer made up of cells called photoreceptors; these cells are sensitive to light.

The macula (about the size of the head of a pin), is a specialized area of the retina containing millions of photoreceptor cells known as cone cells. These function best in bright light levels and allow the person to see fine detail and to recognize colours. The peripheral retina is located away from the central macula, composed primarily of the other photoreceptors called rod cells. These enable us to see when light is dim and provide peripheral vision outside the main line of sight.

When ARMD develops, the cone cells in the macula area become damaged and fail to work as well as they should.

Age-related macular degeneration

Pathophysiology

In the UK, ARMD is the most common cause of irreversible visual loss in those over 50 years. The prevalence of ARMD is increasing in line with an ageing population. Ageing and smoking are the most consistent risk factors for the development of ARMD. Cardiovascular risk factors are also associated with ARMD, with hypertension being a particular risk factor. A positive family history increases the risk. White people are more commonly affected than other ethnic groups.

Age-related macular degeneration (ARMD) is the term given to changes due to ageing occurring without any obvious cause in the macula of people over the age of 50, associated with a chance of loss of vision. This is a disease of the macular area of the retina characterized by the deposition of small colloid bodies (drusen). These are found between the retinal pigment epithelium and the underlying Bruch's membrane, appearing at about the age of 45 years and increasing in size and number. These changes are referred to as age-related maculopathy in the early stages. When they form a critical mass and number in the macular area, ARMD occurs.

Two forms are recognized in late ARMD:
- Atrophic (dry, non-exudative, geographic atrophy): the presence of drusen results in progressive atrophy of the photoreceptors overlying the retinal pigment epithelium and choriocapillaris (underlying the retinal pigment epithelium). This is the most common form of the disease, occurring in 90% of cases.
- Exudative (wet, neovascular): in the remaining 10% of ARMD patients, there is a growth of choroidal vessels under and into the retina, resulting in a neovascular membrane, known as sub-retinal neovascularization. Serous fluid may accumulate here, causing serous retinal detachment. Abnormal vessels may also form over the macula (retinal angiomatous proliferation). Both types of neovascularization result in abnormal vessels that are fenestrated and prone to leakage. The end point of this type of ARMD is scar formation known as disciform macular degeneration.

See Figure 70. 2.

Signs and symptoms

ARMD can be an incidental finding when a person attends a routine visit to the optometrist, especially when only one eye is affected. Some patients may present with difficulty with tasks that require visual discrimination, for example driving, reading and recognizing faces. In the early stages of development of geographic atrophy, diagnosis is often secondary. As the disease progresses, there is a steady decline of central vision that may be associated with distortion of straight lines; micropsia or macropsia can occur. Exudative ARMD is as above, but this may suddenly deteriorate to extreme central vision loss in the event of a bleed. A shower of floaters may precede this.

Examination may uncover a normal or decreased visual acuity. Fundus examination shows discrete yellow deposits in the macular area; these may become paler, larger and confluent in those progressing to exudative ARMD. A bleed may be seen as a dark red, well-defined patch in the macular area. A macular scar may develop: a thick yellow patch over the macular area late in the disease.

Investigations

Slit-lamp examination (bio-microscopy) is required. Optical coherence tomography is often used to support the initial diagnosis and help assess the severity of the disease. This provides the clinician with a cross-sectional view of the retina; the investigation can simply and painlessly be carried out in clinic in a few minutes. Optical coherence tomography is also a useful tool for assessing response to treatment. Those with a suspected neovascular membrane will have fluorescein angiography to assess suitability for treatment. Indocyanine green angiography is sometimes used to provide additional information to fluorescein angiography, this also requires an intravenous injection of a dye.

Management

There are a number of treatments available for wet ARMD. They work by stopping the growth of new blood vessels. Treatment needs to be given quickly once the new blood vessels start. If they are allowed to grow for too long the blood vessels can scar the retina. There is currently no treatment for dry ARMD, as dry ARMD does not involve new blood vessel growth.

Treatment available for wet ARMD is with anti-vascular endothelial growth factor (anti-VEGF). As new blood vessels form in the eye and the body stimulates new blood vessel growth, anti-VEGF drugs interfere with this, preventing vessel growth. By stopping blood vessels growing and leaking, further damage to sight is prevented. An intravitreal injection of anti-VEGF is required. Prior to injection anaesthetic eye drops are given, as well as topical antibiotics; the pupil is dilated. More than one injection of anti-VEGF is usually needed.

Anti-VEGF treatments are usually the first treatment. Photodynamic therapy (PDT) is a type of laser treatment which uses a combination of a light sensitive drug and a low energy laser to stop new blood vessels growing; this is used if anti-VEGF treatment fails.

71 Conjunctivitis

Figure 71.1 The eye and associated structures (the conjunctiva)

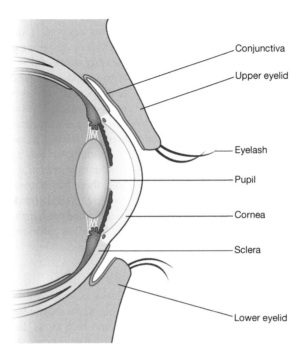

- Conjunctiva
- Upper eyelid
- Eyelash
- Pupil
- Cornea
- Sclera
- Lower eyelid

Figure 71.2 Conjunctivitis

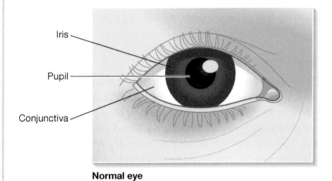

Iris
Pupil
Conjunctiva

Normal eye

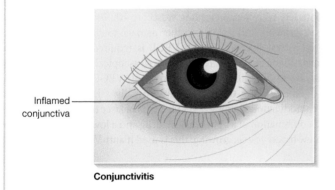

Inflamed conjunctiva

Conjunctivitis

Figure 71.3 Some causes of conjunctivitis

- Viruses
- Bacteria
- Allergies
- A chemical splash in the eye
- A foreign object in the eye
- In newborns, a blocked tear duct

Pathophysiology for Nurses at a Glance, First Edition. Muralitharan Nair and Ian Peate. © 2015 John Wiley & Sons, Ltd. Published 2015 by John Wiley & Sons, Ltd.
Companion website: www.ataglanceseries.com/nursing/pathophysiology

Conjunctivitis

Allergies, viruses or bacteria can cause conjunctivitis (see Figure 71.1). Staphylococci, streptococci, chlamydial organisms and gonococci are common causes of bacterial conjunctivitis. Mild conjunctivitis is generally non-threatening and self-limited. Severe conjunctivitis, for example that caused by gonococci, can result in blindness and can indicate a severe underlying systemic condition.

Pathophysiology

Conjunctivitis refers to inflammation of the conjunctiva. When there is accompanying corneal involvement this gives rise to keratoconjunctivitis, and eyelid involvement points to blepharo-conjunctivitis. Inflammation may be infective or non-infective and can be subdivided further into acute or chronic conjunctivitis. The condition can affect people of any age group, with no gender, ethnic or social discrimination. Generally conjunctivitis is a trivial problem. However, there are occasions when it can lead to permanent or sight-threatening consequences.

The main defence against infection is the epithelial layer covering the conjunctiva. Infection can occur if there is disruption to this barrier.

When infection occurs, the surface tissues of the eye are colonized by normal flora such as streptococci and staphylococci. When alterations occur in the host defence or in the type of bacteria this may lead to clinical infection. Change in the flora can occur by external contamination (e.g. contact lens wear, swimming) or spread from adjacent infectious sites (such as rubbing of the eyes). Figure 71.3 highlights some of the causes of conjunctivitis.

Signs and symptoms

The most common pink eye symptoms include: redness in one or both eyes; itchiness in one or both eyes; a gritty feeling in one or both eyes; discharge in one or both eyes that forms a crust during the night, which can prevent the eye or eyes from opening in the morning; and tearing. The condition is usually generalized, frequently bilateral. Pain is associated with irritation and discomfort; if there is severe pain this suggests something more serious. The presence of photophobia can indicate corneal involvement.

The following may be present: dilated conjunctival vessels (conjunctival injection), conjunctival chemosis (conjunctival oedema), follicles or papillae (see Figure 71.2).

Investigations

A detailed history and examination of the eye(s) is required to help make a diagnosis. It is usual for the diagnosis to be made rapidly after the history and examination have taken place. However, further investigations may be needed and if this is the case the person should be referred to a specialist. Conjunctival scrapings and cultures may be obtained in severe bacterial conjunctivitis or when antibacterial therapy is has been ineffective.

Management

The person should be advised to discontinue contact lens wear until 24–48 hours after resolution of symptoms. Advise the person about taking precautions to reduce transmission of infection, for example no towel or make-up sharing and to avoid rubbing the eyes. The person should return if symptoms worsen within the week or last longer than ten days. Artificial tears may be prescribed to provide comfort and to ease the irritation associated with conjunctivitis.

If the infection is bacterial, antibiotic eye drops may be prescribed, which should eradicate a bacterial infection within several days.

Usually drops are prescribed in preference to ointments. Ointments can be messy and can smear, resulting in blurred vision and for many people this would be impractical. Ointment, however, maintains the concentration of antibacterial medicine in the eye longer than drops and for some people, for example the elderly with poor eye/hand coordination and limited manual dexterity, ointment can be easier to apply. An ideal situation would be to use drops by day and ointment by night.

Bacterial conjunctivitis

Antibiotic eye ointment (chloramphenicol) is sometimes prescribed for treating bacterial conjunctivitis, particularly in children. The ointment may blur vision for up to 20 minutes after application. With both forms of medication, it is expected that signs and symptoms begin to improve in a few days. The antibiotics must be taken for the period prescribed to prevent recurrence of the infection. There is, however, much debate about the use of antibiotics for infective conjunctivitis

Viral conjunctivitis

There is no treatment for most cases of viral conjunctivitis; the infection is usually left to run its own course. Viral conjunctivitis usually begins in one of the eyes and then infects the other eye within a few days. Antiviral medications may be an option if it has been determined that the viral conjunctivitis is caused by the herpes simplex virus. The person should be advised to adhere to strict hygiene measures, such as washing, not sharing towels and not swimming.

Allergic conjunctivitis

Medications that help control allergic reactions, for example antihistamines and mast cell stabilizers, or drugs that help control inflammation, such as decongestants, steroids and anti-inflammatory drops may be prescribed. Avoidance, where possible, of whatever caused the allergies can reduce the severity of the conjunctivitis symptoms.

The management of allergic conjunctivitis is to prevent the release of mediators of allergy, to control the allergic inflammatory cascade and to prevent ocular surface damage that occurs secondary to the allergic response. Cold compresses can be soothing. The use of artificial tears can assist in mild cases; these act to dilute the allergen. To reiterate, contact lenses should not be worn if conjunctivitis is present, or during a course of topical therapy.

Topical ocular antihistamines offer fast relief of the symptoms of allergic conjunctivitis, but they are inappropriate for prolonged use (no longer than six weeks).

Intranasal corticosteroids can reduce ocular symptom, but long-term use can result in cataract, glaucoma and severe bacterial or fungal infections involving the eyelid, conjunctiva and cornea. Oral antihistamines offer relief of symptoms and are useful when the person presents with an associated allergic rhinitis.

Appendix 1: Cross-references to chapters in *Anatomy and Physiology for Nurses at a Glance*

Chapter in *Pathophysiology for Nurses at a Glance*	Relevant chapter in *Anatomy and Physiology for Nurses at a Glance*
Part 1: Pathophysiology	
1. Key principles of pathophysiology	All
2. Cell injury, adaptation and death	All
3. Inflammation, tissue repair and regeneration	All
4. Cancer	Chapters 7 and 20
Part 2: Shock	
5. Cardiogenic shock	Chapter 14
6. Anaphylactic shock	Chapters 3, 5, 7 and 8
7. Hypovolaemic shock	Chapters 2, 3, 5 and 8
8. Septicaemia	Chapters 2, 3, 4, 5 and 6
Part 3: Immunity	
9. Human immunodeficiency virus	Chapter 7
10. Non-Hodgkin lymphoma	Chapter 12
11. Infectious mononucleosis	Chapter 7
Part 4: The nervous system	
12. Meningitis	Chapters 9, 10 and 11
13. Multiple sclerosis	Chapters 9 and 13
14. Parkinson's disease	Chapter 9
15. Cerebrovascular accident	Chapters 9 and 12
Part 5: The blood	
16. Anaemia	Chapter 6
17. Deep vein thrombosis	Chapters 6, 7 and 11
18. Leukaemia	Chapters 6, 7, 8 and 20
19. Thrombocytopenia	Chapters 6, 7 and 8
Part 6: The cardiovascular system	
20. Heart failure	Chapters 14 and 15
21. Myocardial infarction	Chapters 14, 15, 16, 17 and 19
22. Peripheral vascular disease	Chapters 14, 16, 17 and 19
23. Angina	Chapters 14, 15, 16 and 17
Part 7: The respiratory system	
24. Asthma	Chapters 21, 22, 23 and 24
25. Chronic bronchitis	Chapters 21, 22, 23 and 24
26. Pulmonary embolism	Chapters 6, 7, 21, 22, 23 and 24
27. Chronic obstructive pulmonary disease	
Part 8: The gastrointestinal system	
28. Peritonitis	Chapter 26
29. Crohn's disease	Chapters 25 and 26
30. Peptic ulcer	Chapter 25
31. Ulcerative colitis	Chapter 25
32. Bowel cancer	Chapters 25 and 26
Part 9: The hepato-biliary system	
33. Hepatitis	Chapter 27
34. Cholecystitis	Chapters 27 and 28
35. Pancreatitis	Chapter 28
36. Liver cancer	Chapter 27

Pathophysiology for Nurses at a Glance, First Edition. Muralitharan Nair and Ian Peate. © 2015 John Wiley & Sons, Ltd. Published 2015 by John Wiley & Sons, Ltd.
Companion website: www.ataglanceseries.com/nursing/pathophysiology

Chapter in *Pathophysiology for Nurses at a Glance*	Relevant chapter in *Anatomy and Physiology for Nurses at a Glance*
Part 10: The urinary system	
37. Renal failure	Chapters 30, 31 and 33
38. Pyelonephritis	Chapters 30 and 33
39. Renal calculi	Chapters 30, 31 and 33
40. Bladder cancer	Chapter 31
Part 11: The male reproductive system	
41. Benign prostatic hypertrophy	Chapter 35
42. Testicular torsion	Chapter 34
43. Erectile dysfunction	Chapter 34
44. Prostate cancer	Chapter 35
45. Testicular cancer	Chapter 34
Part 12: The female reproductive system	
46. Cancer of the vulva	Chapter 38
47. Menorrhagia	Chapter 40
48. Breast cancer	Chapter 39
49. Cervical cancer	Chapter 37
Part 13: The endocrine system	
50. Diabetes mellitus	Chapters 28, 41 and 43
51. Adrenal insufficiency	Chapter 42
52. Cushing's syndrome	Chapter 42
53. Hyperthyroidism	Chapter 42
Part 14: The musculoskeletal system	
54. Osteoarthritis	Chapters 44, 45, 46 and 47
55. Osteoporosis	Chapters 44, 45, 46 and 47
56. Osteomyelitis	Chapters 44, 45, 46 and 47
57. Gout	Chapter 46
58. Rheumatoid arthritis	Chapters 44, 45, 46 and 47
Part 15: The skin	
59. Atopic dermatitis	Chapter 48
60. Psoriasis	Chapters 48, 50 and 51
61. Acne vulgaris	Chapters 48, 50 and 51
62. Malignant melanoma	Chapters 48, 50 and 51
Part 16: Ear, nose and throat	
63. Otitis media	Chapter 53
64. Ménière's disease	Chapter 53
65. Pharyngitis	Chapters 21 and 54
66. Rhinosinusitis	Chapters 21 and 54
67. Epistaxis	Chapter 54
Part 17: Vision	
68. Cataracts	Chapter 52
69. Glaucoma	Chapter 52
70. Age-related macular degeneration	Chapter 52
71. Conjunctivitis	Chapter 52

Appendix 2: Normal values

Haematology
Full blood count
Haemoglobin (males) 13.0–18.0 g/dL
Haemoglobin (females) 11.5–16.5 g/dL
Haematocrit (males) 0.40–0.52
Haematocrit (females) 0.36–0.47
MCV 80–96 fL
MCH 28–32 pg
MCHC 32–35 g/dL

White cell count 4–11 × 109/L

White cell differential
Neutrophils 1.5–7 × 109/L
Lymphocytes 1.5–4 × 109/L
Monocytes 0–0.8 × 109/L
Eosinophils 0.04–0.4 × 109/L
Basophils 0–0.1 × 109/L

Platelet count 150–400 × 109/L
Reticulocyte count 25–85 × 109/L OR 0.5–2.4%

Erythrocyte sedimentation rate
Westergren
Under 50 years:
Males 0–15 mm/1st hr
Females 0–20 mm/1st hr

Over 50 years:
Males 0–20 mm/1st hr
Females 0–30 mm/1st hr

Plasma viscosity
(25 °C) 1.50–1.72 mPa/s

Coagulation screen
Prothrombin time 11.5–15.5 s
International normalised ratio <1.4
Activated partial thromboplastin time 30–40 s
Fibrinogen 1.8–5.4 g/L
Bleeding time 3–8 m

Coagulation factors
Factors II, V, VII, VIII, IX, X, XI, XII 50–150 IU/dL

Factor V Leiden
Von Willebrand factor 45–150 IU/dL

Von Willebrand factor antigen 50–150 IU/dL
Protein C 80–135 IU/dL
Protein S 80–120 IU/dL
Antithrombin III 80–120 IU/dL
Activated protein C resistance 2.12–4.0
Fibrin degradation products <100 mg/L
D-Dimer screen <0.5 mg/L

Haematinics
Serum iron 12–30 μmol/L
Serum iron-binding capacity 45–75 μmol/L
Serum ferritin 15–300 μg/L
Serum transferrin 2.0–4.0 g/L
Serum B12 160–760 ng/L
Serum folate 2.0–11.0 μg/L
Red cell folate 160–640 μg/L
Serum haptoglobin 0.13–1.63 g/L

Haemoglobin electrophoresis
Haemoglobin A >95%
Haemoglobin A2 2–3%
Haemoglobin F <2%

Chemistry
Serum sodium 137–144 mmol/L
Serum potassium 3.5–4.9 mmol/L
Serum chloride 95–107 mmol/L
Serum bicarbonate 20–28 mmol/L
Anion gap 12–16 mmol/L
Serum urea 2.5–7.5 mmol/L
Serum creatinine 60–110 μmol/L
Serum corrected calcium 2.2–2.6 mmol/L
Serum phosphate 0.8–1.4 mmol/L
Serum total protein 61–76 g/L
Serum albumin 37–49 g/L
Serum total bilirubin 1–22 μmol/L
Serum conjugated bilirubin 0–3.4 μmol/L
Serum alanine aminotransferase 5–35 U/L
Serum aspartate aminotransferase 1–31 U/L
Serum alkaline phosphatase 45–105 U/L (over 14 years)
Serum gamma glutamyl transferase 4–35 U/L (<50 U/L in males)
Serum lactate dehydrogenase 10–250 U/L
Serum creatine kinase (males) 24–195 U/L
Serum creatine kinase (females) 24–170 U/L

Pathophysiology for Nurses at a Glance, First Edition. Muralitharan Nair and Ian Peate. © 2015 John Wiley & Sons, Ltd. Published 2015 by John Wiley & Sons, Ltd.
Companion website: www.ataglanceseries.com/nursing/pathophysiology

Creatine kinase MB fraction <5%
Serum troponin I 0–0.4 µg/L
Serum troponin T 0–0.1 µg/L
Serum copper 12–26 µmol/L
Serum caeruloplasmin 200–350 mg/L
Serum aluminium 0–10 µg/L
Serum magnesium 0.75–1.05 mmol/L
Serum zinc 6–25 µmol/L
Serum urate (males) 0.23–0.46 mmol/L
Serum urate (females) 0.19–0.36 mmol/L
Plasma lactate 0.6–1.8 mmol/L
Plasma ammonia 12–55 µmol/L
Serum angiotensin-converting enzyme 25–82 U/L
Fasting plasma glucose 3.0–6.0 mmol/L
Haemoglobin A1 C 3.8–6.4%
Fructosamine <285 µmo/L
Serum amylase 60–180 U/L
Plasma osmolality 278–305 mosmol/kg

Lipids and lipoproteins

The target levels will vary depending on the patient's overall cardiovascular risk assessment.
Serum cholesterol: <5.2 mmol/L
Serum LDL cholesterol: <3.36 mmol/L
Serum HDL cholesterol: >1.55 mmol/L
Fasting serum triglyceride 0.45–1.69 mmol/L

Blood gases (breathing air at sea level)

Blood H + 35–45 nmol/L
pH 7.36–7.44
PaO2 11.3–12.6 kPa
PaCO2 4.7–6.0 kPa
Base excess ±2 mmol/L

Carboxyhaemoglobin

Non-smoker <2%
Smoker 3–15%

Immunology/rheumatology

Complement C3 65–190 mg/dL
Complement C4 15–50 mg/dL

Total haemolytic (CH50) 150–250 U/L
Serum C-reactive protein <10 mg/L

Serum immunoglobins

IgG 6.0–13.0 g/L
IgA 0.8–3.0 g/L
IgM 0.4–2.5 g/L
IgE <120 kU/L
Serum β2 micro globulin <3 mg/L

Cerebrospinal fluid

Opening pressure 50–180 mm H_2O
Total protein 0.15–0.45 g/L
Albumin 0.066–0.442 g/L
Chloride 116–122 mmol/L
Glucose 3.3–4.4 mmol/L
Lactate 1–2 mmol/L
Cell count ≤5 mL-1
Differential:
Lymphocytes 60–70%
Monocytes 30–50%
Neutrophils none
IgG/ALB ≤0.26
IgG index ≤0.88

Urine

Glomerular filtration rate 70–140 mL/min
Total protein <0.2 g/24 h
Albumin <30 mg/24 h
Calcium 2.5–7.5 mmol/24 h
Urobilinogen 1.7–5.9 µmol/24 h
Coproporphyrin <300 nmol/24 h
Uroporphyrin 6–24 nmol/24 h
Delta-aminolevulinate 8–53 µmol/24 h
5-hydroxyindoleacetic acid 10–47 µmol/24 h
Osmolality 350–1000 mosmol/kg

Faeces

Nitrogen 70–140 mmol/24 h
Urobilinogen 50–500 µmol/24 h
Fat (on normal diet) <7 g/24 h

Appendix 3: Prefixes and suffixes

Prefix: A prefix is positioned at the beginning of a word to modify or change its meaning. Pre means 'before'. Prefixes may also indicate a location, number, or time.

Suffix: The ending part of a word that changes the meaning of the word.

Prefix or suffix	Meaning	Example(s)
a-, an-	not, without	analgesic, apathy
ab-	from, away from	abduction
abdomin(o)-	of or relating to the abdomen	abdomen
acous(io)-	of or relating to hearing	acoumeter, acoustician
acr(o)-	extremity, topmost	acrocrany, acromegaly, acroosteolysis, acroposthia
ad-	at, increase, on, toward	adduction
aden(o)- aden(i)-	of or relating to a gland	adenocarcinoma, adenology, adenotome, adenotyphus
adip(o)-	of or relating to fat or fatty tissue	adipocyte
adren(o)-	of or relating to adrenal glands	adrenal artery
-aemia	blood condition	anaemia
aer(o)-	air, gas	aerosinusitis
aesthes-	sensation	anaesthesia
alb-	denoting a white or pale colour	albino
alge(si)-	pain	analgesic
-algia, alg(i)o-	pain	myalgia
all(o-)	denoting something as different, or as an addition	alloantigen, allopathy
ambi-	denoting something as positioned on both sides, describing both of two	ambidextrous
amni-	pertaining to the membranous foetal sac (amnion)	amniocentesis
an-	not, without	analgesia
ana-	back, again, up	anaplasia
andr(o)-	pertaining to a man	android, andrology
angi(o)-	blood vessel	angiogram
ankyl(o)-, ancyl(o)-	denoting something as crooked or bent	ankylosis
ante-	describing something as positioned in front of another thing	antepartum
anti-	describing something as 'against' or 'opposed to' another	antibody, antipsychotic
arteri(o)-	of or pertaining to an artery	arteriole, artery
arthr(o)-	of or pertaining to the joints, limbs	arthritis
articul(o)-	joint	articulation
-ase	enzyme	lactase
-asthenia	weakness	myasthenia gravis
ather(o)-	fatty deposit, soft gruel-like deposit	atherosclerosis
atri(o)-	an atrium (esp. heart atrium)	atrioventricular
aur(i)-	of or pertaining to the ear	aural
aut(o)-	self	autoimmune
axill-	of or pertaining to the armpit (uncommon as a prefix)	axilla
bi-	twice, double	binary
bio-	life	biology
blephar(o)-	of or pertaining to the eyelid	blepharoplast
brachi(o)-	of or relating to the arm	brachium of inferior colliculus
brady-	'slow'	bradycardia

Pathophysiology for Nurses at a Glance, First Edition. Muralitharan Nair and Ian Peate. © 2015 John Wiley & Sons, Ltd. Published 2015 by John Wiley & Sons, Ltd.
Companion website: www.ataglanceseries.com/nursing/pathophysiology

Prefix or suffix	Meaning	Example(s)
bronch(i)-	bronchus	bronchiolitis obliterans
bucc(o)-	of or pertaining to the cheek	buccolabial
burs(o)-	bursa (fluid sac between the bones)	bursitis
carcin(o)-	cancer	carcinoma
cardi(o)-	of or pertaining to the heart	cardiology
carp(o)-	of or pertaining to the wrist	carpopedal
-cele	pouching, hernia	hydrocele, varicocele
-centesis	surgical puncture for aspiration	amniocentesis
cephal(o)-	of or pertaining to the head (as a whole)	cephalalgy
cerebell(o)-	of or pertaining to the cerebellum	cerebellum
cerebr(o)-	of or pertaining to the brain	cerebrology
chem(o)-	chemistry, drug	chemotherapy
chol(e)-	of or pertaining to bile	cholecystitis
cholecyst(o)-	of or pertaining to the gall bladder	cholecystectomy
chondr(i)o-	cartilage, gristle, granule, granular	chondrocalcinosis
chrom(ato)-	colour	haemochromatosis
-cidal, -cide	killing, destroying	bacteriocidal
cili-	of or pertaining to the cilia, the eyelashes; eyelids	ciliary
circum-	denoting something as 'around' another	circumcision
col-, colo-, colono-	colon	colonoscopy
colp(o)-	of or pertaining to the vagina	colposcopy
contra	against	contraindicate
coron(o)-	crown	coronary
cost(o)-	of or pertaining to the ribs	costochondral
crani(o)-	belonging or relating to the cranium	craniology
-crine, crin(o)	to secrete	endocrine
cry(o)-	cold	cryoablation
cutane-	skin	subcutaneous
cyan(o)-	denotes a blue colour	cyanopsia
cycl-	circle, cycle	cyclodialysis
cyst(o)-, cyst(i)-	of or pertaining to the urinary bladder	cystotomy
cyt(o)-	cell	cytokine
-cyte	cell	leukocyte
-dactyl(o)-	of or pertaining to a finger, toe	dactylology, polydactyly
dent-	of or pertaining to teeth	dentist
dermat(o)- derm(o)-	of or pertaining to the skin	dermatology
-desis	binding	arthrodesis
dextr(o)-	right, on the right side	dextrocardia
di-	two	diplopia
dia-	through, during, across	dialysis
dif-	apart, separation	different
digit-	of or pertaining to the finger (rare as a root)	digit
-dipsia	suffix meaning (condition of) thirst	polydipsia, hydroadipsia, oligodipsia
dors(o)-, dors(i)-	of or pertaining to the back	dorsal, dorsocephalad
duodeno-	duodenum, twelve: upper part of the small intestine (twelve inches long on average), connects to the stomach	duodenal atresia
dynam(o)-	force, energy, power	hand strength dynamometer
-dynia	pain	vulvodynia
dys-	bad, difficult, defective, abnormal	dysphagia, dysphasia
ec-	out, away	ectopia, ectopic pregnancy
ect(o)-	outer, outside	ectoblast, ectoderm
-ectasia, -ectasis	expansion, dilation	bronchiectasis, telangiectasia
-ectomy	denotes a surgical operation or removal of a body part, resection, excision	mastectomy
-emesis	vomiting condition	haematemesis
-aemia	blood condition	anaemia
encephal(o)-	of or pertaining to the brain, also see cerebro	encephalogram
endo-	denotes something as 'inside' or 'within'	endocrinology, endospore
eosin (o)-	red	eosinophil granulocyte
enter(o)-	of or pertaining to the intestine	gastroenterology

Prefix or suffix	Meaning	Example(s)
epi-	on, upon	epicardium, epidermis, epidural, episclera, epistaxis
erythr(o)-	denotes a red colour	erythrocyte
ex-	out of, away from	excision, exophthalmos
exo-	denotes something as 'outside' another	exoskeleton
extra-	outside	extradural haematoma
faci(o)-	of or pertaining to the face	facioplegic
fibr(o)-	fibre	fibroblast
fore-	before or ahead	foreword
fossa-	a hollow or depressed area; trench or channel	fossa ovalis
front-	of or pertaining to the forehead	frontonasal
galact(o)-	milk	galactorrhoea
gastr(o)-	of or pertaining to the stomach	gastric bypass
-genic	formative, pertaining to producing	cardiogenic shock
gingiv-	of or pertaining to the gums	gingivitis
glauc(o)-	denoting a grey or bluish-grey colour	glaucoma
gloss(o)-, glott(o)-	of or pertaining to the tongue	glossology
gluco-	sweet	glucocorticoid
glyc(o)-	sugar	glycolysis
-gnosis	knowledge	diagnosis, prognosis
gon(o)-	seed, semen, also reproductive	gonorrhoea
-gram, -gramme	record or picture	angiogram
-graph	instrument used to record data or picture	electrocardiograph
-graphy	process of recording	angiography
gyn(aec)o-	woman	gynaecomastia
halluc-	to wander in mind	hallucinosis
haemat-, haemato- (haem-)	of or pertaining to blood	haematology
haemangi-, haemangio-	blood vessels	haemangioma
hemi-	one-half	cerebral hemisphere
hepat- (hepatic-)	of or pertaining to the liver	hepatology
heter(o)-	denotes something as 'the other' (of two), as an addition, or different	heterogeneous
hist(o)-, histio-	tissue	histology
home(o)-	similar	homeopathy
hom(o)-	denotes something as 'the same' as another or common	homosexuality
hydr(o)-	water	hydrophobe
hyper-	denotes something as 'extreme' or 'beyond normal'	hypertension
hyp(o)-	denotes something as 'below normal'	hypovolemia,
hyster(o)-	of or pertaining to the womb, the uterus	hysterectomy, hysteria
iatr(o)-	of or pertaining to medicine, or a physician	iatrogenic
-iatry	denotes a field in medicine of a certain body component	podiatry, psychiatry
-ics	organized knowledge, treatment	obstetrics
ileo-	ileum	ileocecal valve
infra-	below	infrahyoid muscles
inter-	between, among	interarticular ligament
intra-	within	intramural
ipsi-	same	ipsilateral hemiparesis
ischio-	of or pertaining to the ischium, the hip-joint	ischioanal fossa
-ism	condition, disease	dwarfism
-ismus	spasm, contraction	hemiballismus
iso-	denoting something as being 'equal'	isotonic
-ist	one who specializes in	pathologist
-itis	inflammation	tonsillitis
-ium	structure, tissue	pericardium
juxta (iuxta)	near to, alongside or next to	juxtaglomerular apparatus
karyo-	nucleus	eukaryote
kerat(o)-	cornea (eye or skin)	keratoscope

Prefix or suffix	Meaning	Example(s)
kin(e)-, kin(o), kinaesi(o)-	movement	kinaesthesia
kyph(o)-	humped	kyphoscoliosis
labi(o)-	of or pertaining to the lip	labiodental
lacrim(o)-	tear	lacrimal canaliculi
lact(i)-, lact(o)	milk	lactation
lapar(o)-	of or pertaining to the abdominal wall, flank	laparotomy
laryng(o)-	of or pertaining to the larynx, the lower throat cavity where the voice box is	laryngeal oedema
latero-	lateral	lateral pectoral nerve
-lepsis, -lepsy	attack, seizure	epilepsy, narcolepsy
lept(o)-	light, slender	leptomeningeal
leuc(o)-, leuk(o)-	denoting a white colour	leukocyte
lingu(a)-, lingu(o)-	of or pertaining to the tongue	linguistics
lip(o)-	fat	liposuction
lith(o)-	stone, calculus	lithotripsy
log(o)-	speech	logogram
-logist	denotes someone who studies a certain field	oncologist, pathologist
-logy	denotes the academic study or practice of a certain field	haematology, urology
lymph(o)-	lymph	lymphoedema
lys(o)-, -lytic	dissolution	lysosome
-lysis	destruction, separation	paralysis
macr(o)-	large, long	macrophage
-malacia	softening	osteomalacia
mamm(o)-	of or pertaining to the breast	mammogram
mammill(o)-	of or pertaining to the nipple	mammillaplasty, mammillitis
manu-	of or pertaining to the hand	manufacture
mast(o)-	of or pertaining to the breast	mastectomy
meg(a)-, megal(o)-, -megaly	enlargement, million	splenomegaly, megameter
melan(o)-	black colour	melanin
mening(o)-	membrane	meningitis
meta-	after, behind	metacarpus
-meter	instrument used to measure or count	sphygmomanometer
-metry	process of measuring	optometry
metr(o)-	pertaining to conditions or instruments of the uterus	metrorrhagia
micro-	denoting something as small, or relating to smallness, millionth	microscope
milli-	thousandth	millilitre
mon(o)-	single	infectious mononucleosis
morph(o)-	form, shape	morphology
muscul(o)-	muscle	musculoskeletal system
my(o)-	of or relating to muscle	myoblast
myc(o)-	fungus	onychomycosis
myel(o)-	of or relating to bone marrow or spinal cord	myeloblast
myri-	ten thousand	myriad
myring(o)-	eardrum	myringotomy
narc(o)-	numb, sleep	narcolepsy
nas(o)-	of or pertaining to the nose	nasal
necr(o)-	death	necrosis, necrotizing fasciitis
neo-	new	neoplasm
nephr(o)-	of or pertaining to the kidney	nephrology
neur(i)-, neur(o)-	of or pertaining to nerves and the nervous system	neurofibromatosis
normo-	normal	normocapnia
ocul(o)-	of or pertaining to the eye	oculist
odont(o)-	of or pertaining to teeth	orthodontist
odyn(o)-	pain	stomatodynia
-oesophageal, oesophago-	gullet	oesophagus
-oid	resemblance to	sarcoidosis
-ole	small or little	bronchiole
olig(o)-	denoting something as 'having little, having few'	oliguria

Prefix or suffix	Meaning	Example(s)
-oma (singular) **-omata** (plural)	tumour, mass, collection	sarcoma, teratoma
onco-	tumour, bulk, volume	oncology
onych(o)-	of or pertaining to the nail (of a finger or toe)	onychophagy
oo-	of or pertaining to the an egg, a woman's egg, the ovum	oogenesis
oophor(o)-	of or pertaining to the woman's ovary	oophorectomy
ophthalm(o)-	of or pertaining to the eye	ophthalmology
optic(o)-	of or relating to chemical properties of the eye	opticochemical, biopsy
orchi(o)-,orchid(o)-,orch(o)-	testis	orchiectomy, orchidectomy
-osis	a condition, disease or increase	harlequin type ichthyosis, psychosis, osteoperosis
osseo-	bony	osseous
ossi-	bone	peripheral ossifying fibroma
ost(e)-, oste(o)-	bone	osteoporosis
ot(o)-	of or pertaining to the ear	otology
ovo-, ovi-, ov-	of or pertaining to the eggs, the ovum	ovogenesis
oxo-	addition of oxygen	oxygenate

Prefix or suffix	Meaning	Example(s)
pachy-	thick	pachyderma
palpebr-	of or pertaining to the eyelid (uncommon as a root)	palpebra
pan-, pant(o)-	denoting something as 'complete' or containing 'everything'	panophobia, panopticon
papill-	of or pertaining to the nipple (of the chest/breast)	papillitis
papul(o)-	indicates papulosity, a small elevation or swelling in the skin, a pimple, swelling	papulation
para-	alongside of, abnormal	paracyesis
-paresis	slight paralysis	hemiparesis
parvo-	small	parvovirus
path(o)-	disease	pathology
-pathy	denotes (with a negative sense) a disease, or disorder	sociopathy, neuropathy
pector-	breast	pectoralgia, pectoriloquy, pectorophony
ped-, -ped-, -pes	of or pertaining to the foot, -footed	pedoscope
paed-, paedo-	of or pertaining to the child	paediatrics. paedophilia
pelv(i)- pelv(o)-	hip bone	pelvis
-penia	deficiency	osteopenia
-pepsia	denotes something relating to digestion, or the digestive tract	dyspepsia
peri-	denoting something with a position 'surrounding' or 'around' another	periodontal
-pexy	fixation	nephropexy
phaco-	lens-shaped	phacolysis, phacometer, phacoscotoma
-phage -phagia	forms terms denoting conditions relating to eating or ingestion	sarcophagia
-phago-	eating, devouring	phagocyte
phagist-	forms nouns that denote a person who 'feeds on' the first element or part of the word	lotophagi
-phagy	forms nouns that denotes 'feeding on' the first element or part of the word	haematophagy
pharmaco-	drug, medication	pharmacology
pharyng(o)-	of or pertaining to the pharynx, the upper throat cavity	pharyngitis, pharyngoscopy
phleb(o)-	of or pertaining to the (blood) veins, a vein	phlebography, phlebotomy
-phobia	exaggerated fear, sensitivity	arachnophobia
phon(o)-	sound	phonograph, symphony
phos-	of or pertaining to light or its chemical properties, now historic and used rarely; see the common root phot(o)- below	phosphene
phot(o)-	of or pertaining to light	photopathy
phren(i)-, phren(o)-, phrenico	the mind	phrenic nerve, schizophrenia, diaphragm
-plasia	formation, development	achondroplasia
-plasty	surgical repair, reconstruction	rhinoplasty
-plegia	paralysis	paraplegia
pleio-	more, excessive, multiple	pleiomorphism
pleur(o)-, pleur(a)	of or pertaining to the ribs	pleurogenous
-plexy	stroke or seizure	cataplexy

Prefix or suffix	Meaning	Example(s)
pneum(o)-	of or pertaining to the lungs	pneumonocyte, pneumonia
pneumat(o)-	air, lung	pneumatic
-poiesis	production	haematopoiesis
poly-	denotes a 'plurality' of something	polymyositis
post-	denotes something as 'after' or 'behind' another	postoperation, post-mortem
pre-	denotes something as 'before' another (in (physical) position or time)	premature birth
presby(o)-	old age	presbyopia
prim-	denotes something as 'first' or 'most-important'	primary
proct(o)-	anus, rectum	proctology
prot(o)-	denotes something as 'first' or 'most important'	protoneuron
pseud(o)-	denotes something false or fake	pseudoephedrine
psych(e)-, psych(o)	of or pertaining to the mind	psychology, psychiatry
psor-	itching	psoriasis
-ptosis	falling, drooping, downward placement, prolapse	apoptosis, nephroptosis
-ptysis	(a spitting), spitting, haemoptysis, the spitting of blood derived from the lungs or bronchial tubes	haemoptysis
pulmon-, pulmo-	of or relating to the lungs	pulmonary
pyel(o)-	pelvis	pyelonephritis
py(o)-	pus	pyometra
pyr(o)-	fever	antipyretic
quadr(i)-	four	quadriceps
radio-	radiation	radiowave
ren(o)-	of or pertaining to the kidney	renal
retro-	backward, behind	retroversion, retroverted
rhin(o)-	of or pertaining to the nose	rhinoceros, rhinoplasty
rhod(o)-	denoting a rose-red colour	rhodophyte
-rrhage	burst forth	haemorrhage
-rrhagia	rapid flow of blood	menorrhagia
-rrhaphy	surgical suturing	aortorrhaphy
-rrhexis	rupture	karyorrhexis
-rrhoea	flowing, discharge	diarrhoea
-rupt	break or burst	erupt, interrupt
salping(o)-	of or pertaining to tubes, e.g. Fallopian tubes	salpingectomy, salpingopharyngeus muscle
sangui-, sanguine-	of or pertaining to blood	sanguine
sarco-	muscular, fleshlike	sarcoma
scler(o)-	hard	scleroderma
-sclerosis	hardening	atherosclerosis, multiple sclerosis
scoli(o)-	twisted	scoliosis
-scope	instrument for viewing	stethoscope
-scopy	use of instrument for viewing	endoscopy
semi-	one-half, partly	semiconscious
sial(o)-	saliva, salivary gland	sialagogue
sigmoid(o)-	sigmoid, s-shaped curvature	sigmoid colon
sinistr(o)-	left, left side	sinistrotorsion
sinus-	of or pertaining to the sinus	sinusitis
somat(o)-, somatico-	body, bodily	somatic
-spadias	slit, fissure	hypospadias, epispadias
spasmo-	spasm	spasmodic dysphonia
sperma-, spermo-, spermato-	semen, spermatozoa	spermatogenesis
splen(o)-	spleen	splenectomy
spondyl(o)-	of or pertaining to the spine, the vertebra	spondylitis
squamos(o)-	denoting something as 'full of scales' or 'scaly'	squamous cell
-stalsis	contraction	peristalsis
-stasis	stopping, standing	cytostasis, homeostasis
-staxis	dripping, trickling	epistaxis
sten(o)-	denoting something as 'narrow in shape' or pertaining to narrowness	stenography
-stenosis	abnormal narrowing in a blood vessel or other tubular organ or structure	restenosis, stenosis

Prefix or suffix	Meaning	Example(s)
stomat(o)-	of or pertaining to the mouth	stomatogastric, stomatognathic system
-stomy	creation of an opening	colostomy
sub-	beneath	subcutaneous tissue
super-	in excess, above, superior	superior vena cava
supra-	above, excessive	supraorbital vein
tachy-	denoting something as fast, irregularly fast	tachycardia
-tension, -tensive	pressure	hypertension
tetan-	rigid, tense	tetanus
thec-	case, sheath	intrathecal
therap-	treatment	hydrotherapy, therapeutic
therm(o)-	heat	thermometer
thorac(i)-, thorac(o)-, thoracico-	of or pertaining to the upper chest, chest; the area above the breast and under the neck	thorax
thromb(o)-	of or relating to a blood clot, clotting of blood	thrombus, thrombocytopenia
thyr(o)-	thyroid	thyroid
thym-	emotions	dysthymia
-tome	cutting instrument	dermatome
-tomy	act of cutting; incising, incision	gastrotomy
tono-	tone, tension, pressure	tonometry
top(o)-	place, topical	topical anesthetic
tort(i)-	twisted	torticollis
tox(i)-	toxin, poison	toxoplasmosis
tox(o)-		
toxic(o)-		
trache(a)-	trachea	tracheotomy
trachel(o)-	of or pertaining to the neck	tracheloplasty
trans-	denoting something as moving or situated 'across' or 'through'	transfusion
tri-	three	triangle
trich(i)-	of or pertaining to hair, hair-like structure	trichocyst
trichia		
trich(o)-		
-tripsy	crushing	lithotripsy
-trophy	nourishment, development	pseudohypertrophy
tympan(o)-	eardrum	tympanocentesis
-ula, -ule	small	nodule
un(i)-	one	unilateral hearing loss
ur(o)-	of or pertaining to urine, the urinary system; (specifically) pertaining to the physiological chemistry of urine	urology
uter(o)-	of or pertaining to the uterus or womb	uterus
vagin-	of or pertaining to the vagina	vagina
varic(o)-	swollen or twisted vein	varicose
vas(o)-	duct, blood vessel	vasoconstriction
vasculo-	blood vessel	vasculopathy
ven-	of or pertaining to the (blood) veins, a vein (used in terms pertaining to the vascular system)	vein, venospasm
ventr(o)-	of or pertaining to the belly; the stomach cavities	ventrodorsal
ventricul(o)-	of or pertaining to the ventricles; any hollow region inside an organ	cardiac ventriculography
-version	turning	anteversion, retroversion
vesic(o)-	of or pertaining to the bladder	vesical arteries
viscer(o)-	of or pertaining to the internal organs, the viscera	viscera
xanth(o)-	denoting a yellow colour, an abnormally yellow colour	xanthopathy
xen(o)-	foreign, different	xenograft
xer(o)-	dry, desert-like	xerostomia
zo(o)-	animal, animal life	zoology
zym(o)-	fermentation	enzyme, lysozyme

Appendix 4: Glossary of terms

Acquired an acquired disorder is a medical condition which develops post-foetally

Acute of sudden onset

Aetiology the study of the cause of a disease

Aggregate the clumping together in the blood

Agonist a substance that acts like another substance and therefore stimulates an action

Allergen substance that can produce hypersensitivity reactions in the body

Anaphylaxis a severe, systemic allergic response characterized by vasodilation and bronchoconstriction

Anoxia total depletion of oxygen

Antigens substances (often proteins) causing formation of an antibody that reacts specifically with that antibody

Aplastic anaemia disease in which the bone marrow, and the blood stem cells that reside there, are damaged, resulting in reduced blood cells

Apoptosis a process of programmed cell death

Arteries blood vessels that transport blood away from the heart

Ascites the build-up of fluid in the space between the lining of the abdomen and abdominal organs (the peritoneal cavity)

Atheromatous plaques a deposit or degenerative accumulation of lipid-containing plaques on the innermost layer of the wall of an artery

Atrophy decrease in size

Autoimmune An autoimmune disorder is a condition that occurs when the immune system mistakenly attacks and destroys healthy body tissue

Azotaemia see uraemia

Basophils a type of white blood cell

Benign a non-malignant neoplasm

Blebbing protrusions of the cell membrane

Boas' sign the presence of an area of hyperaesthesia at the site of radiation of the pain to the back, typically below the scapula

Brudzinski's sign flexion of the neck that causes hip and knee to flex

Calculi stones

Capillaries small blood vessels where exchange between blood and the tissue cells takes place

Carcinogens cancer causing substances

Carcinoma a malignancy originating in epithelial tissues

Cardiac output volume of blood pumped out every minute by the ventricle

Chronic a disease developing gradually lasting longer than three months

Cilia hair-like projections that sweep dust and other foreign particles out

Colonoscope an examination that views the inside of the colon (large intestine) and rectum, using a tool called a colonoscope

Congenital a condition existing at birth and often before birth

Coronary revascularization the restoration of perfusion to the coronary arteries as a result of ischaemia

Cyanosis blue discolouration, usually of the lips and fingers

Cytotoxic drugs chemotherapy drugs

Defaecate to pass stool (motion)

Demyelination to destroy or remove the myelin sheath of (a nerve fibre), as through disease

Diaphoresis excessive sweating

Dyspnoea difficulty in breathing

Eclampsia seizures (convulsions) in a pregnant woman, not related to an existing brain condition

Engulfing swallowing up

Enzymes are biological catalysts – catalysts are substances that increase the rate of chemical reactions without being used up

Enzymes proteins that speed up chemical reactions in a cell

Eosinophils a type of white blood cell

Epigastric relating to the abdominal region lying between the hypochondriac regions and above the umbilical region

Erythropoietin a hormone that stimulate the production of red blood cells in the bone marrow

Exacerbation an increase in the severity of a disease or any of its signs or symptoms

Fatigue extreme tiredness

Fibrinogen a protein in the blood plasma that is essential for the coagulation of blood and is converted to fibrin by the action of thrombin in the presence of ionized calcium

Fistula an abnormal connection between an organ, vessel, or intestine and another structure

Genetics concerns the process of trait inheritance from parents to offspring

Genotoxic pertaining to agents known to damage DNA, thereby causing mutations, which can result in cancer

Goblet cells glandular epithelial cells found in the lining of the digestive and respiratory tracts that secrete mucus

Haemopoiesis the formation of blood cells in the living body (especially in the bone marrow)

Hemiparesis weakness

Hydronephrosis a condition where one or both kidneys become stretched and swollen as a result of a build up of urine inside the kidney(s)

Hypercalcaemia high levels of calcium in the blood

Hyperkalaemia high levels of potassium in the blood

Hyperplasia increase in cell number

Hypertrophy to increase in size

Hypersensitivity reaction an altered immunological response to an antigen resulting in a pathological immune response upon re-exposure

Hypoalbuminaemia a medical condition where levels of albumin in blood serum are abnormally low

Hypocellular containing less than the normal number of cells

Hypoglycaemia low blood glucose

Hypokalaemia low levels of potassium in the blood

Hyponatraemia low levels of sodium in the blood

Hypoperfusion decreased blood flow through an organ, as in hypovolemic shock; if prolonged, it may result in permanent cellular dysfunction and death

Pathophysiology for Nurses at a Glance, First Edition. Muralitharan Nair and Ian Peate. © 2015 John Wiley & Sons, Ltd. Published 2015 by John Wiley & Sons, Ltd.
Companion website: www.ataglanceseries.com/nursing/pathophysiology

Hypoxaemia a lower than normal oxygen content of the blood as measured in an arterial blood sample

Idiopathic having no demonstrable cause

Immunoglobulins antibodies

Immune response a defence function of the body that produces antibodies to destroy invading antigens and malignancies

Immunosuppressants powerful medicines that dampen down the activity of the body's immune system

Inflammation swelling

Inflammatory response tissue reaction to injury or to an antigen; can include pain, swelling, itching, redness, heat and loss of function

Inotrope a drug that alters the force or energy of muscular contractions

Integrin transmembrane receptor that mediates the attachment between a cell and its surroundings, such as other cells or the extracellular matrix

Ischaemia insufficient perfusion of oxygenated blood to a body organ or part

Kernig's sign inability to extend the knee while the hip is flexed at a 90-degree angle

Kinin polypeptide hormones that are formed locally in the tissues and cause dilation of blood vessels and contraction of smooth muscle

Lethargy lack of energy

Macrophages a cell which ingests and destroys microbrs and foreign matter

Malaise a vague feeling of bodily discomfort, as at the beginning of an illness

Malignant a cancerous neoplasm

Mast cells a cell found in the connective tissue that releases histamine during inflammation

Mesothelial cells a membrane that forms the lining of several body cavities the pleura, peritoneum and pericardium

Mesothelial tissue also surrounds the male internal reproductive organs and covers the internal reproductive organs of women

Metaplasia reversible replacement of one mature cell type by another less mature type

Metastasise spread of the tumour cells

Microemboli tiny blood clots

Mucoprotein any of a group of organic compounds, such as the mucins, that consist of a complex of proteins and glycosaminoglycans and are found in body tissues and fluids

Murphy sign elicited by firmly placing a hand at the costal margin in the right upper abdominal quadrant and asking the patient to breathe deeply; if the gall bladder is inflamed, the patient will experience pain and catch their breath as the gall bladder descends and contacts the palpating hand

Mutation altered or changed

Necrosis death of cells or tissues through injury or disease, especially in a localized area of the body

Negative feedback mechanisms mechanisms that usually result in a response that balances a change in system

Neoplasia growth of cells and tissue into new areas, resulting in a tumour; can be benign or malignant

Nucleation is the process where droplets of liquid can condense from a vapour, or bubbles of gas can form in a boiling liquid

Oesophagus gullet

Oligodendrocytes myelin producing cells

Orthostasis maintenance of an upright standing posture

Pancytopenia a medical condition in which there is a reduction in the number of red and white blood cells, as well as platelets

Pathogenesis events leading to the development of a disease and the signs and symptoms occurring as the disease progresses

Pathology the study of changes in cell/tissue structure related to disease or death

Pathophysiology the study of the disturbance of normal mechanical, physical and biochemical functions, either caused by a disease, or resulting from a disease or abnormal syndrome or condition that may not qualify to be called a disease

Petechiae pinpoint-sized reddish-purple spots on the skin

Petechial rashes small spots

Phagocytes white blood cells

Phagocytose to envelop and destroy bacteria and other foreign material

Photophobia aversion to light

Pluripotent capable of differentiating into one of many cell types

Polyps small growths on the inner lining of the colon

Proctitis inflammation of the rectum

Pyuria pus in the urine

Reticulin a scleroprotein from the connective fibres of reticular tissue

Sclera the white of the eye

Selectins a family of cell adhesion molecules

Septicaemia blood infection

Serosal a serous membrane, especially one that lines the pericardial, pleural and peritoneal cavities, enclosing their contents

Shock a condition of severely inadequate blood flow to the body's peripheral tissues, associated with life-threatening cellular dysfunction; also known as hypoperfusion

Sigmoidoscope a procedure used to see inside the sigmoid colon and rectum

Sinusoids small blood vessels, similar to capillaries

Stenosis narrowing of any canal or opening, for example the intestine, a blood vessel or a heart valve

Supersaturation to cause (a chemical solution) to be more highly concentrated than is normally possible under given conditions of temperature and pressure

Systemic a condtion that affects the entire body

Tachycardia rapid heart rate

Tachypnoes rapid breathing

Thromboxane a substance made by platelets that causes blood clotting and constriction of blood vessels

Tinnitus the perception of a noise in one or both ears, for example a ringing in the ears

Trigone a smooth triangular area on the inner surface of the bladder limited by the apertures of the ureters and urethra

Uraemia the accumulation of waste products, normally excreted in the urine, in the blood causes severe headaches, vomiting, etc.

Urethral sphincter one of two muscles used to control the exit of urine in the urinary bladder through the urethra

Vasculitis inflammation of the wall of a blood vessel

Venules small veins

Wheezing a coarse whistling sound produced when airways are partially obstructed

Further reading

Booth, K. (2013) *Anatomy, Physiology and Disease for the Health Professions*, 3e. McGraw-Hill, New York.

Braun, C. (2011) *Pathophysiology: A Clinical Approach*. Lippincott, Baltimore.

Copstead, L.E. (2010) *Pathophysiology*, 4e. Elsevier, St Louis.

Gould, B.E. (2011) *Study Guide for Pathophysiology for the Health Professions*, 4e. Elsevier, St Louis.

Huether, S.E., McCance, K.L., Brashers, V.L. & Rote, N.S. (2010) *Pathophysiology: The Biologic Basis for Disease in Adults and Children*, 6e. Elsevier, St Louis.

Huether, S.E., McCance, K.L., Brashers, V.L. & Rote, N.S. (2012) *Understanding Pathophysiology*, 5e. Elsevier, St Louis.

Nair, M. & Peate, I. (2013) *Fundamentals of Applied Pathophysiology: An Essential Guide for Nursing and Healthcare Students*, 2e. Wiley, Oxford.

Peate, I. & Nair, M. (2015) *Anatomy and Physiology for Nurses at a Glance*. Wiley, Oxford.

Pathophysiology for Nurses at a Glance, First Edition. Muralitharan Nair and Ian Peate. © 2015 John Wiley & Sons, Ltd. Published 2015 by John Wiley & Sons, Ltd.
Companion website: www.ataglanceseries.com/nursing/pathophysiology

Index

Pathophysiology for Nurses at a Glance, First Edition. Muralitharan Nair and Ian Peate. © 2015 John Wiley & Sons, Ltd. Published 2015 by John Wiley & Sons, Ltd.
Companion website: www.ataglanceseries.com/nursing/pathophysiology